BODY MANDALA

"Mary Bond's book *Body Mandala* is her latest compendium of self-guided somatic education tools. This book was well worth the wait. Mary has given us more than fifty years of her teachings, meticulously researched through her work with many clients and movement professionals. I cannot recommend this book highly enough. It is the perfect toolkit for anyone who wants to get rid of self-imposed limitations and discover new ways to move."

STACY BARROWS, PT, DPT, GCFP, PMA-CPT, INVENTOR,
AUTHOR OF *THE SMARTROLLER GUIDE,* AND DIRECTOR
OF CENTURY CITY PHYSICAL THERAPY

"Mary has the impressive ability to write clearly and succinctly while also drawing the reader to connect inside themselves using bodily sensing exercises, metaphor, and story. I was inspired to engage in each of the somatic exercises as I read through the chapters of *Body Mandala;* as I did so, I was reminded of how easy it is to ignore certain areas of the body and certain kinds of aches and imbalances. Mary's somatic practices are simple yet take one to a deep place of inner attention. Engaging in the exercises, I was also reminded of the importance of taking the time to deeply perceive and lovingly care for this precious body. The practices in this book have profound implications for awareness and health."

CYNTHIA PRICE, PH.D., LMT, RESEARCH PROFESSOR IN
THE DEPARTMENT OF BIOBEHAVIORAL NURSING AT THE UNIVERSITY OF
WASHINGTON AND DIRECTOR OF THE CENTER FOR MINDFUL BODY AWARENESS

"Mary Bond's work is a light of clarity in the field of movement and embodiment. In *Body Mandala* she shares with the reader and practitioner an invitation to explore one's knowing and being. Mary Bond is a living presence who has weaved her own experience, teaching, and knowledge into an exquisite work of art in embodiment. As such, her book is required curriculum in our Structural Integration program at the University of New Mexico–Taos. It is the foundational approach we use in our movement and embodiment training. Her book is an inspiration for the first-time layperson wanting to begin a practice in embodiment and teaches those with more experience in the field how to teach embodiment. She brings clear examples of fascial anatomy, creating ground and support through one's system and open curiosity to explore oneself in living presence."

KIRSTIE SEGARRA, PH.D., SOMATIC MEDICINE PRACTITIONER,
DOCTOR OF INTEGRATIVE MEDICINE,
AND BOARD CERTIFIED STRUCTURAL INTEGRATOR

"Depth. Clarity. Simplicity. These three words describe the magic of this book, which uncovers secrets of a life in which incarnation can become joyous. With a maturity that is rare in the study of gesture and in writing, Mary Bond makes it possible to take a path, which she maps out so well, to a movement practice that can beautify our lives."

HUBERT GODARD, PH.D., ROLF MOVEMENT PRACTITIONER
AND CERTIFIED ROLFER

"When artisans distill their lived experience into form, an unmistakable resonance happens. Whether the medium is the written word, a practice, a painting, really any act of creation, their lived experience sounds a gong within us. It evokes a quickening of sorts, an impulse to be more deeply embodied. Mary Bond is that sort of artisan: she has spent more than seven decades in a love affair with the lived experience of being in a body. We can feel and taste this extraordinary love infused in every word, idea, and practice in her book."

BO FORBES, PSY.D., YOGA, MINDFULNESS, AND
EMBODIMENT EDUCATOR AND AUTHOR OF
YOGA FOR EMOTIONAL BALANCE

"I view this book as a true investment in the journey to whole body health, an investment in body, mind, and future. The whole body concept introduces the new scientific foundation with related anatomy concepts and function in easy-to-digest language and order. Illustrations and video guide you into the related embodied movement skills. I gladly recommend Mary's enlightening body of work for the movement professional and anyone in pursuit of a better body. A must-do book to always have by my side."

MARIE-JOSÉ BLOM-LAWRENCE, PILATES MASTER TEACHER,
MOVEMENT EDUCATOR, AND INTERNATIONAL PRESENTER

"Mary Bond has, once again, succeeded in showing us new ways to understand and practice healthy movement, this time including additional connections to our thoughts and psyche. *Body Mandala* stimulates my curiosity and gets me excited to apply the practices to my own work as a choreographer and dance educator."

RUTH BARNES, CHOREOGRAPHER, DANCER,
AND PROFESSOR AND DANCE PROGRAM COORDINATOR AT
MISSOURI STATE UNIVERSITY

"*Body Mandala* acts not only as a beautiful field guide to your body as a continuous whole, but also contains the kind of guided movement and awareness explorations that only a true master can articulate. In short, Mary Bond has written a book that is not only a cognitive game changer regarding how we understand our bodies but is also a somatic and experiential guide to coming deeply home to your own body."

BROOKE THOMAS, SOMATIC EDUCATOR

BODY MANDALA

Posture, Perception, and Presence

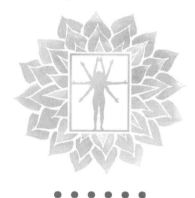

• • • • • •

MARY BOND

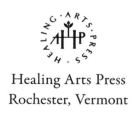

Healing Arts Press
Rochester, Vermont

Healing Arts Press
One Park Street
Rochester, Vermont 05767
www.HealingArtsPress.com

Healing Arts Press is a division of Inner Traditions International

Note to the reader: This book is intended as an informational guide. The remedies, approaches, and techniques described herein are meant to supplement, and not to be a substitute for, professional medical care or treatment. They should not be used to treat a serious ailment without prior consultation with a qualified health care professional.

Cataloging-in-Publication Data for this title is available from the Library of Congress

ISBN 978-1-64411-882-5 (print)
ISBN 978-1-64411-883-2 (ebook)

Printed and bound in the United States by P. A. Hutchison Company

10   9   8   7   6   5   4   3   2   1

Text design and layout by Virginia Scott Bowman
This book was typeset in Garamond Premier Pro with Nexa used as the display typeface

To send correspondence to the author of this book, mail a first-class letter to the author c/o Inner Traditions • Bear & Company, One Park Street, Rochester, VT 05767, and we will forward the communication, or contact the author directly at **healyourposture.com**.

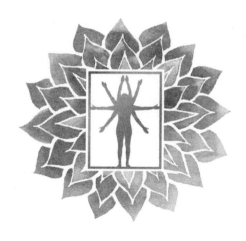

CONTENTS

PART 3

Practicing

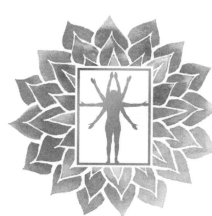

EXPLORATIONS AND PRACTICES

Audio and Video Instruction

🔊 To access the exercises shared in this book, please visit
audio.innertraditions.com/bodman

PART 1
. . . .
Orienting

PART 2
· · · · · · · · · · · · · ·
Deepening

PART 3

Practicing

FOREWORD

By Thomas Myers

Mary Bond is the genuine article. In the world of "bodywork," a young science with a high turnover rate of "facts," there are always fads arising and then fading, each of which contain a grain of truth, but lack sufficient coherence to endure.

The book you are holding is not part of a fad. It is deep, persuasive, well grounded, and poetic—not in the sense of being fanciful, but in the sense of resonance with the many levels on which a real life is lived.

In terms of our bodies, there are two trends afloat in the world today. On the one hand, advertising, convenience, and an increasingly automated society have produced an "inactivity crisis" that has increasingly separated humans from their "felt sense," their kinesthetic awareness.

The poet Juvenal coined *mens sana in corpore sano*—a healthy mind needs a healthy body—back in the Roman times, but it applies today in spades. Too many of our children graduate high school knowing more about social media than they know about the most intimate and proximate tool they will ever have—their miraculous bodies. This leads to a loss not only of physical health and abilities but also mental alertness and intuitive skills. Not to mention lost days at work from avoidable injuries.

The opposing trend is the revivification of the body through movement, integrative manual therapy, and awareness practice. This trend is developing quickly but still involves only a small percentage of the population. When I was young, yoga was unheard of; now a wide variety of yoga styles are available in every town, nearly on every corner. Likewise, the advances in personal training, Pilates, Feldenkrais, dance, and a hundred other somatic practices.

Any movement is better than no movement, but better still is an inclusive movement program that runs—as this book does—from stillness (that is a movement, too) to vigorous exercise, with special attention to the daily "diet" of movement—walking, reaching, sitting, and lifting—that occupy most of us for most of the time.

That is what you will find here. Mary's diverse and extensive experience allows her to navigate the complex topography of kinesthetic experience with a deft confidence. Neither the philosophy, insights, or exercises in this book will be replaced next year with some bright new thing—this book will stand the test of time.

Coupled with the electronic supplemental material that she has prepared, Mary's new and long-awaited book, like a mandala, stretches out with applications in all the directions of your inner compass from the mundane to the extraordinary.

Your body is part of your spiritual life, as well as your biomechanical and bio-emotional life. "Occupying Your Body" is just as important (and more readily available) as occupying Wall Street. Fully inhabiting your body is a political and environmental act, not just a self-help health project.

Mary Bond's practices are practical and expansive, specific and inclusive, well founded in biology, and yet touching the feeling sides where we all live. Awareness determines the quality of life, and Mary is a master facilitator of awareness.

Read the book—it is a joy—but more importantly, take on the practices Mary puts forward here.

THOMAS MYERS, AUTHOR OF *ANATOMY TRAINS*
CLARKS COVE, MAINE
APRIL 2017

The originator of the Anatomy Trains Myofascial Meridians, THOMAS MYERS studied with Ida Rolf, Moshe Feldenkrais, and Buckminster Fuller, and with a variety of movement and manual therapy pioneers. His work is influenced by cranial, visceral, and intrinsic movement studies he made with European schools of osteopathy. An inveterate traveler, Tom has practiced integrative manual therapy for over forty years in a variety of clinical and cultural settings. Tom is the author of *Anatomy Trains* (2020, 4th ed), coauthor of *Fascial Release for Structural Balance* (2010, 2017), coauthor of *Anatomy Trains in Motion Study Guide* (2019), author of *Body3, The Anatomist's Corner, Structural Integration: Collected Articles,* and *BodyReading: Visual Assessment and the Anatomy Trains,* and has also written extensively for *Journal of Bodywork and Movement Therapies.* He has also produced over twenty online learning courses with Anatomy Trains, and others in collaboration with various body-oriented professional groups. Tom lives and sails on the coast of Maine in the USA. Tom and his faculty conduct professional development courses and certification in Structural Integration worldwide.

PREFACE

It has been my experience that people who understand and respect their bodies tend to have an open and compassionate perspective on life. My mission, as a writer, teacher, and Rolfing Structural Integration practitioner is to help people further that understanding and respect. I believe that becoming more attuned to our body awareness affects the choices we make in relation to ourselves, to our fellow human beings, to our environment, and to our planet. My mission, then, is to contribute to humanity's deeper embodiment.

This book shares harvest from my nearly fifty years' involvement in various mind-body pursuits. It contains techniques, exercises, and ways of experiencing my body that I've learned from others or have developed myself, that I teach to clients and students, and that I practice for my own benefit. It's my hope that these gleanings will benefit you as well—that they will help you fend off suggestions that your body is merely decorative or only a vehicle for your mind.

Conscious embodiment helps us become more perceptive beings. *Body Mandala* expresses my somatic philosophy—my belief that our bodies are the means for understanding the fundamental nature of existence. I see this philosophy as a way to help save our planet.

I hope that it will not take as long for you as it did for me to inhabit the glory of your body.

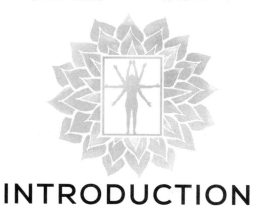

INTRODUCTION

What Is a Body Mandala?

Embodiment as a Practice

I've been a student of the human body ever since putting on my ballet shoes at age six. In the beginning my interest was driven by aesthetics, by the wish to perform well and to appear attractive. Twenty years later, this interest led me to become a practitioner of Structural Integration, a form of bodywork developed by Ida P. Rolf, Ph.D., that is dedicated to restoring the body's optimal posture and movement. As a bodyworker, I applied the knowledge I'd sought for my own benefit to help other people improve their postures and reduce posture-related pain.

In time, performing this service taught me that there is more to posture than meets the eye. Obvious in hindsight, but primed by my culture, it took a disconcertingly long time for this basic truth to sink in. Mainstream American culture, a powerful hypnotic force, is obsessed with bodily appearance. So, at the outset of my career, I focused on helping people stand straighter and move more gracefully. In time I saw that better posture and movement were not sustainable unless they became by-products of embodiment.

Embodiment is the process of awakening to the grace and wisdom of your body. Body awareness is the key to that awakening. Each of our bodies is a receptacle of precious and inimitable history, each one unique, and each one replete with exquisite sensory intelligence. Learning to tap into that intelligence changes how it feels to be alive. That difference in feeling transforms posture and movement.

Transforming your body involves an inner journey that is more like a meditation practice than a route you can plan with a GPS. Each person's travels are unique. The map for your journey of embodiment *is* your body with all its activities—your sense of balance and alignment, your habitual movements, your perceptions, emotions, and attitudes.

Like a mandala, a visual image used to focus the mind in certain meditative disciplines, your body contains an intricate network of pathways and intersections that lead to your most loving and gracious sense of aliveness—to your best self. Your body, in and of itself, becomes your practice. Because your personal Body Mandala is always present, you can be engaged with it at any moment of your day. Such self-study may yield profound spiritual insights, help you manifest your talents, alert you to unbeneficial beliefs, and coach you to "be at your best" at any moment. It also improves your posture.

Any meditation practice increases your capacity to quiet the mental mono-logue that yanks awareness between past and future. The "be here now" message keeps finding new iterations as the Digital Age relentlessly pushes our attention out of the present and into the next moment, and the next, and the next. There is nothing more "here and now" than your own body. Building the habit of body awareness helps anchor you in the present.

Mandalas

The word "mandala" derives from an ancient Sanskrit word meaning "container of essence." It commonly refers to a pattern of visual images that represents the relationship between our inner and outer worlds. Mandala designs are rendered in various media, including paint, cloth, and sand. In most traditions, a circle is bounded by a square with four entry points or "gates" that lead to a central image. The central figure represents the goal of the practice—self-realization or enlightenment.

Mandalas have appeared through many historical periods and in many cultures. All represent the human journey to self-understanding. In Hindu and Buddhist spiritual traditions, mandalas are used to focus attention during meditation. Christian symbols, such as halos and circular stained-glass windows, are similar to mandalas in both outer form and inner meaning—as guidance for the progression from the material world to the divine inner center. Judaism prohibits visual images of a deity but incorporates mandala-like concepts such as the Tree of Life centrally placed in the Garden of Eden. In Islam, the structure of the mosque can be seen as a mandala with the dome of the roof representing the heavens. Native American medicine wheels also embrace a mandala pattern.

In the modern era, psychoanalyst Carl Jung described the spontaneous circle drawings that both he and his patients made as mandalas. He believed the doodles were part of the process of harmoniously integrating one's personality.

REFLECTION
Good Morning, Sensei

Behind the closed door, Sensei begins his morning mantra. It's uncanny how he knows my eyes have opened. He chants boldly for several refrains and then, thankfully, he pauses.

Lying spread-eagled, appreciating the quiet, I twist my torso and legs to one side and then the other, testing how it feels to be alive today.

Sensei, louder now, resumes his chanting: "Eeoooow. Meeooow!"

Apart from his fixation on food, my cat, Sensei, is a mellow soul. I chose his name—"Teacher"—to remind myself to surrender petty irritations like the sound of his voice. That's easier some mornings than others. Today I'm rushing through the bathroom and onward through the house, my mental beeline on the cat food shelf. Only food will shut him up.

Stumbling into the kitchen, my body awareness is left behind on the bed. By ignoring the stiffness that is a natural result of eight hours of inactivity, I've succumbed to it. I shuffle my feet like a wooden old lady.

I know my body to be otherwise. As a septuagenarian I can forgive myself for being creaky in the morning. But I also know that moving stiffly—ambulating with the bare minimum of joints engaged—becomes a habit that can't be blamed entirely on my bodily tissues. Habits take place in the brain. The more frequently I move stiffly, the more familiar and less optional that way of moving becomes.

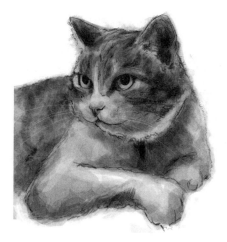

I can choose how I move. I slow down. I manage to tune out the cat.

Ah, now I can call up a walking rhythm that evokes resilience in my body. I choose to feel my body's weight and substance. I remind my soles to sense the floor; remind my ankles and toes to bend. It feels better now—that little "give" to my footsteps loosens up my hips.

The morning light streaming in through the windows sparks my peripheral vision. My narrowed, defensive perspective softens. There's a hummingbird in the oak tree, and a tender wind strokes the bamboo chimes. My chest uncoils and I inhale. Much better. I choose to open my body to the day.

Relax, Sensei. Your food is coming.

Your Body as a Mandala

In *The New Rules of Posture,* I explained that some people habitually orient to the present moment by grounding themselves, while others seek support by scanning their spatial surroundings. Both of these perceptual orientations are healthy and necessary. In certain situations, the best response is to hold one's ground, whereas in other situations, it is wise to run away. Too much spatial orientation can make fleeing the scene—physically or metaphorically—a habitual response. Too much ground orientation inclines one to intransigence. In *The New Rules,* I proposed that healthy posture manifests when we have both perceptual orientations simultaneously and are free to move between them as situations demand.

My *New Rules* message is a simplified rendering of a broader philosophy and model of the ways in which the brain organizes human movement. This model is the work of French movement theorist Hubert Godard. His work has been incorporated into the curriculum of the Rolf Institute of Structural Integration, where I taught for many years.

When I was first exposed to Godard's theory, I entered a classroom to see it diagramed on a white board in the form of a circle with a highlighted central area and four points of entry. This was exciting to me because although I had always been interested in human movement, I had never been presented with a satisfying way to codify it. At the time, I didn't identify the chart as a mandala, although now that seems obvious. I've spent more than two decades practicing this movement theory in my life and sharing my version of it with others. It is the basis of the practice I'm proposing in this book and the inspiration for my coinage of the phrase Body Mandala.

The central focus of Godard's model is what he calls "tonic function."[1] The word **tonic** refers to a type of muscular response. Tonic muscles are equipped, through their relationships with the circulatory, nervous, and connective tissue systems, to be capable of sustained contraction. Their partners, the **phasic** muscles, receive nutrients and neural signals differently and are geared for shorter bursts of effort. Long-distance runners rely on their tonic muscles; sprinters have well-developed phasic muscles.

The sustained and mostly unconscious activity of your tonic muscles helps keep you upright. Not only that, but your tonic system, which includes parts of your brain and nervous system, actually acts *before* you move to orient your body to the situation at hand. Your body orients to the sound of your phone's beep a nanosecond before you reach for it.

This means that posture is not only a stacking up of parts but is also a dynamic perceptual activity. It is your immediate response to what's going on around you.

Your tonic function, then, describes your way of being in the world, your embodied presence. This pertains to your physical stance but also to your mental and emotional attitudes and points of view. It's a product of the activities of your nerves, muscles, and the connective tissues that pervade your entire body. Because the tonic system is ordered deep within unconscious parts of the brain, it's impossible to authentically and sustainably change your being through conscious acts of will. Your presence does change, however, through four distinct influences. These influences are akin to the entry points or gates portrayed in traditional mandalas.

Posture

One point of access to your embodied presence is your habitual posture—how you stand. This is your structural alignment and balance. It includes the tensional relationships between your bones, muscles, and the connective tissues that compose your body's shape. Bodywork that is strategic to structural organization can help alter postural form, but form also changes through influences coming in via the other gates.

Sensation

A second access point is the information that comes into your body through your senses, as well as sensations that occur within your body. Over 80 percent of the nervous system is involved in processing or organizing sensory input, so, in a way, your body is mainly a sensory processing module.

Your sense perceptions are usually paired with a movement response that in turn affects your postural alignment and balance. In this way the three "gates" of movement,

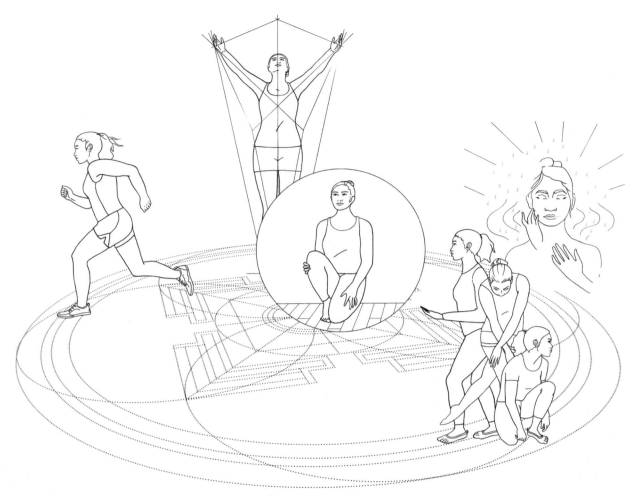

Your somatic presence is accessible through the gates of posture, sensation, movement, and expression.

posture, and sensation all affect each other and contribute to how you express yourself in the world. This process was the main topic of *The New Rules of Posture.*

Movement

Movement is your third entry point. Your every movement is coordinated by your nervous system. This includes your respiration, digestion, and heartbeat, the way you walk and bend over, the way you wave, smile, or frown. Much of your coordination is learned, like chewing, speaking, or riding a bicycle, although some movements, like the urge to breathe, or an infant's sucking reflex, are "hardwired." To a vast degree, your coordination is so unconscious that you take it for granted. Walking on two legs is an incredibly intricate coordinative feat that you mastered long ago and no longer think much about.

But not having to think about moving has a downside. Since life in the twenty-first century doesn't demand much variety of movement, or, in fact, much movement at all, our bodies become less and less versatile. The automatic movements that make up your daily grind can keep you in a rut that degrades your posture over time. Reduced movement can even sully your perceptions and affect how you interact with other people. What occurs in any one region of your Body Mandala affects all the other areas.

Expression

Expression, the fourth entry point, includes all your work and play, your emotion and communication. It includes your obvious ways of expressing yourself, like speaking, dancing, or shooting hoops. What may be less obvious is that you express yourself in the way you walk, even in the way you breathe.

Your habitual ways of expressing yourself connect to all the other gates, as well as to your embodied presence at the center of the mandala. For example, a period of psychotherapy that brings about increased self-confidence, contentment, or openness can change the way you stand and move and amplify your receptivity to new sensations and perceptions. Learning a new skill—perhaps studying a martial art—involves you in a new repertoire of sensation and movement that can transform both your postural organization and the confidence with which you communicate with others.

Limited expression, such as an occupation that confines you to a forty-hour week of sitting and repetitive movement adversely affects your posture, lessens your capacity to move your body in innovative ways, and limits your perception of your surroundings. This can affect self-expression in many ways. Absent healthy self-expression, some people withdraw, or act outrageously or aggressively. Others are drawn into addictions, straying ever further from authentic presence. How you inhabit your Body Mandala has social consequences.

Somatic Presence

"Soma" comes from a Greek word that indicates a living body. In conventional medicine, the word "somatic" refers to the body as distinct from mind or spirit. Among bodyworkers, movement teachers, and alternative medicine practitioners, somatic also connotes the subjective, conscious experience of being present in your body.

The central figure in a traditional mandala represents enlightenment or access to the divine. The central figure in your Body Mandala is your embodied, or somatic, presence. Essential to your presence are two distinct sensory experiences—perceptions of wholeness and of physical centeredness.

Current scientific research into the body's connective tissues—collectively known as **fascia**—supports the view that wholeness is a physical, felt experience. Formerly assumed to be mere packing material for muscles, bones, and organs, scientists now regard fascia as the fundamental ingredient of living beings. It is a continuous, uninterrupted webbing—something like a sea sponge—that is present everywhere in the body. Significantly, fascia has been found to be replete with sensory nerves. We know ourselves as whole beings thanks to the sensory signals within our fascia. Your Body Mandala journey will involve learning more about fascia and tapping into this previously unknown organ of your body.

Your sense of centeredness is distilled in your body's midline. A central vertical line is the conventional way to represent a body's relationship to gravity. But gravity is only one of many forces that organize our bodies. Perceptual orientation—how we gauge our safety with respect to our surroundings—is also an organizing element. Perception of a threat compresses or twists the midline; exuberance lifts and lengthens it. Further, the human midline is an embryonic expression of aliveness that is manifest in our tissues long before we must orient ourselves in the world. We are born knowing center.

Being present in the moment—the aim of many forms of meditation—has been shown to improve mental and physical health.[2] My premise in *Body Mandala* is that cultivating somatic presence contributes to the same ends. It also complements a dedicated meditation practice if you're already involved in one.

Posture is an entryway to somatic presence. Because posture is most likely something you're already concerned about, it can become an incentive for developing the awareness you need to be fully present in your body on a daily basis. But this involves some self-study.

Tracking my sensations, stances, gestures, moods, and behaviors has been a way to learn about myself. Paying attention to my bodily experience has given me a measure of choice about how I live from moment to moment. What I learned as a movement theory became a map for tracing my personal journey. The objective of Godard's model is a body that acts gracefully and efficiently under stress and is adaptable to any context. Applied to the whole person, this means to be alive in your whole being and present to all that happens.

For me that includes being open, generous, and resilient. But desirable qualities of presence are as variable as the sky: serenity and exuberance, power and tenderness, fury and sorrow. You need to be present in all kinds of ways in this increasingly complicated and uncertain world. If you can be centered and whole in your body, any emotional expression can be incorporated into your kaleidoscope of presence.

The Present

Consider times when you've accidentally hurt yourself—banged your head on an open cupboard door, tripped over an electric cord, or bathed your eyes with make-up remover instead of eye drops. In the nanoseconds before those things occurred, you weren't present in your body. You were neither grounded, nor aware of your surroundings. You were mentally out in front of, or far behind, your body's current experience.

The Dalai Lama is said to have observed: "There are only two days in the year that nothing can be done. One is called yesterday and the other is called tomorrow." Why is it so difficult for us to heed this obvious truth?

Aging

Along with the importance of being present, I also want to consider the future—your future. The fact that bodies age is something few people under the age of thirty-five consider to be applicable to themselves. I was well into my fifties before I fully grasped this truth. At a certain moment I realized that I had become irrelevant to mainstream values and trends—I had become an elder.

This will happen to you. Bodies inevitably age, no matter how technologically and cosmetically adept we may become at staving off the process.

As a septuagenarian, I'm well aware that my time left here is far less than I've lived. But I've been fortunate to have a calling that has required embodiment and self-care. When I look around at my aging contemporaries, I observe that bodies that have been taken for granted stiffen up and break down more readily than those that have been respectfully tended. I'm sad to see my friends feeling surprised and offended when their bodies begin to fail. Of course, genetics plays a part, as do diet and lifestyle. And none of us knows what waits around the corner. But it's worth considering that the practice of embodiment may provide a hedge against the stiffening, bending, and closing of the physical aging process.

How This Book Is Organized

Body Mandala is a study guide for your personal mandala journey. The presentation includes concepts and ideas to think about in tandem with sensations and emotions to feel. Somatic practices and meditations are presented in the accompanying audio and video files. These are my attempts to communicate as directly as I can with your body. Some of the recorded meditations have a hypnotic quality, so please do not play them while driving or operating other machinery.

What I'm trying to share with you will make the most sense if you do the physical practices whenever you see the audio or video icon 🔊. These are available at **audio.innertraditions.com/bodman**.

Boxed sections are "scripts" for the audio and video files. Most of these passages are intentionally repetitive and slow-paced, more like guided meditations than exercise instructions. For anyone who would like to share the experiences with others, having access to these scripts should make it easy. Read them slowly, with pauses between the sentences. Let the words sink in.

In part 1—"Orienting," I introduce basic information about fascia and about how your brain organizes movement and sensation. Then I present fundamental concepts that support embodied presence and explorations that promote it.

In part 2—"Deepening," I offer exploratory practices designed to develop your experience of somatic wholeness and of your midline. You'll also deepen your understanding of posture by questioning the commonly accepted premise that having good posture is like aligning a stack of blocks. You'll learn about and begin to experience the body-organizing principle of **tensegrity**—the multidimensioned, integrated tensioning of your body's fascia. You'll also glance at science that supports the idea that refined body awareness is both normal and practical. The section concludes with an extended journey through your spine.

Part 3—"Practicing," considers how the sedentary, electronic era in which we live affects our bodies and suggests ways to navigate between embodied experience and the increasingly disembodying experience of living in a technology-centered world. Books are linear constructions with numerically ordered chapters. But because deep body learning is not a linear process, my presentation is somewhat spiralic. You'll meet some ideas again and again, experiencing them more profoundly with each circuit. I want your Body Mandala experience to be as physical as possible, so I've tried to place experiential material ahead of discussion. That way you'll feel what I'm talking about before trying to understand it.

The New Rules of Posture

In *The New Rules of Posture,* I wrote about posture as perceptual activity. I defined posture as the small and usually unnoticed movements we make to orient ourselves to situations, emotions, and relationships with others. In that book I proposed six body "zones" that help create postural improvements: the pelvic floor, the breathing muscles, the abdomen, the hands and shoulders, the feet, and the head. The book included self-care exercises that enable healthy function in each zone, along with basic ergonomic information and case histories. *Body Mandala* builds on the premise that posture is perceptual orientation. Rather than repeat extensive discussions of breathing and of abdominal and shoulder support, I refer the reader to the earlier volume for more on those topics.

Somatic Contemplations

The word "exercise" connotes an activity that involves physical effort in order to increase strength and stamina. Exercising implies work, as in "working out." This mode of training often regards the body as an enemy or naughty child that must be made to mend her ways. Such treatment can make us detach from the experience, just as a punished child would do. It's ironic that time spent improving the body often results in disembodying experiences.

In contrast, somatic contemplations in this book focus on ways for you to become more present in your physical experience. They attune you to your current physical habits and bring awareness to sensations in your body that you haven't noticed or valued before. Introspective in approach, they require your full attention. It will be important to set aside practice time when you won't be interrupted, and also to choose a setting that feels private and safe.

By practicing the somatic contemplations, your ability to concentrate on them deepens in quality and lengthens in time. This deepening lets your brain develop new neural connections. Once these connections are established, you feel more balanced and aligned, more efficient and graceful as you move, and more freely expressive in your body. Conversely, rote repetition of a practice, like a mindlessly chanted mantra, will bring you nothing new.

The Body Mandala practices will not make you stronger or more flexible, and none of them is a quick fix for posture or movement problems. All of them will affect your awareness and coordination and contribute to your sense of wholeness and midline—to your presence. What I'm sharing here is a body philosophy that can serve you for a lifetime.

Many of the practices show you different perspectives of the same somatic lessons. My intention is to help you cumulatively build an experience of your body as whole cloth. I want to help you embody the principle of tensegrity thoroughly enough that it becomes a new way of being in your body. When that happens, you'll know organically how to incorporate your Body Mandala practice into other body disciplines, into artistic or athletic endeavors, and into your daily life.

If the approach feels insufficiently vigorous or insufficiently social for you, try to stick with it long enough to feel something new in your body. Later on, this inner work will yield surprising improvements in performance of any activity—golf, horseback riding, tango, tennis, kettlebells, or gardening.

REFLECTION
First Love

Tommy delivered papers in my neighborhood before school. Each morning his fat bicycle tires skidded to a stop outside the window where I sat practicing piano. When I'd turn around to look, he'd wink and take off down the street. I wrote his initials on the soles of my shoes.

I can still see Tommy's big old grin and the blond peach fuzz on his Adam's apple. In the way of ten-year-old boys, he mimicked how I walked. Evidently I held my left arm close to my chest, elbow bent, and wrist dangling. He made it look strange. In the way of ten-year-old girls, I found this both infuriating and titillating.

That odd arm and shoulder habit has been a lifelong feature of my Body Mandala, appearing, disappearing, returning in disguise, and leading me on a goose chase of self. I've explored it from the perspective of posture, as an imbalance in my shoulder girdle. But I knew it also as a movement—an incipient wincing gesture that I've learned to sense even when my arm is hanging straight down. It was an expression of little Mary Bond walking to school. What did it feel like in those days? What perception underlays its origin? Was there a specific event that set it off? Can I know? Do I need to know?

Walking as Integration

I suggest that you walk around for a few minutes after experiencing each of the somatic contemplations. Locomotion helps your brain integrate new sensations, gradually altering your coordination and your expression. Integration is the most important phase in any of the practices. Sensation by sensation, you'll be developing options for the way you move through your life.

Find a place to walk where you have room to move freely, a space of at least thirty feet. Walk at a comfortable pace and allow your arms to swing.

When you stride down a long hallway, or better yet, along a park path, your tissues expand and recoil, imparting suppleness to your steps. When you walk short distances, stopping and starting, your muscles work harder because there's not enough room for full expansion of your connective tissues. James Earls, author of *Born to Walk,* calls this "museum walking." It tires you out.

Reflections

Throughout the book I've shared some of my own somatic experiences. I want to demonstrate that perfectly mundane experiences may contribute to the kinds of sensory and expressive "aha's" that are found through somatic contemplation. Current culture invites us to place more value on dramatic experiences than on prosaic ones. But we are all essentially and equally pedestrian. A quiet epiphany can sometimes have more lasting impact on your self-understanding than an explosion of awareness.

A Little Science

Interspersed between the theory and experiential work are short discussions of scientific findings that will ground your body awareness in real world data. You'll learn about your body-wide network of fascia, about the neural plasticity of your brain, and about the fabulous vagus nerve that oversees well-being of both body and mind. These topics will support your experience of your body as a profoundly inter-communicative organism and lead you to value body awareness as both practical and health giving.

> ### Tibetan Sand Mandalas
>
> Tibetan monks spend many days creating intricate mandalas of colored sand. After prayers and devotions, the sand is swept up and poured into a lake or river to circulate the mandala's creative energy.
>
> Like sand mandalas, our bodies, too, will be swept away. It is said that the depth of the journey will lighten the sweeping.

Glossary

Somatic movement education, like any field, has its own nomenclature. Words that might not be familiar to a general reader are defined, usually the first time they're used, and are marked in bold in the running text. You'll find a glossary (p. 255) for easy reference as you move through the book.

Practical Somatic Literacy

Body Mandala is about the practical value of sensing your body. Your body awareness is your "somatic literacy." By refining it you gain:

- Improved posture, which contributes positively to your appearance and diminishes posture-related pain.
- More efficient and more graceful movement.
- Increased self-understanding and clearer intuition.
- A way to prevent stress reactions from taking over your day.

All of this affects the way you travel through your life and, therefore, also affects the way you age.

Body Mandala practice can touch you in ways that "shake your tree" emotionally. Although somatic literacy can aid in resolving psychological issues, it is not a substitute for working with a therapist. An internet search can help you find a somatic or body-oriented psychotherapist.

PART 1
Orienting

Chapter 1 introduces you to your organ of embodiment, your fascia. The burgeoning research about the nature of this tissue is changing the way I conceive of my body and understand its intelligence. I'm eager to share this perspective with you.

Beginning in chapter 2, you'll explore your orienting perceptions. First, you'll discover that your perception of being supported by the ground depends on your experience of your bodily weight. After that, you'll investigate ways in which your awareness of space—within and outside your body—also contributes to your experience of feeling supported.

The human significance of ground and space is not a novel concept. Prophets and yogis have spoken of humanity's equilibrium between heaven and earth for eons. You already know that your feet are on the ground, and that to get anything done, you must move through space. But savoring these perceptions, fully tasting the ways in which they serve you, helps you realize the degree to which you've taken them for granted. Diminished perceptions of the ground and of your spatial surroundings lessen your ability to cope with things—to balance and to respond with efficiency, ease, and grace. Simple awareness of these two orienting perceptions contributes to a fuller sense of being present, here and now, in three-dimensional, grounded wholeness.

Body Reading

To receive the full impact of the somatic practices in this book, it will be helpful to establish a baseline for your awareness. In the series of assessments that follow, you'll have the opportunity to notice basic details about your alignment, your body sensations, your coordination and movement, and your self-expression. You'll be observing yourself through each mandala gate. Anchor what you learn by keeping a journal while you work your way through this book. Make a few notes about what you feel during the body reading. It's a preliminary map of your Body Mandala. In chapter 2, you'll start filling in more details.

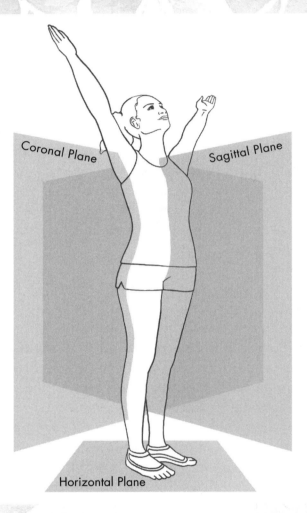

Coronal Plane

Sagittal Plane

Horizontal Plane

Sagittal *comes from the same root as Sagittarius, the astrological archer whose arrow flies straight ahead. The sideways plane is called the **coronal plane,** from corona, the halo around the moon, or around images of holy figures. The vertical line where the two planes intersect is a common measure of stationary body alignment. The **horizontal plane,** relating to the horizon, is perpendicular to the body's central vertical line.*

Stance and Structure

🔊 Practice 1 - Stance and Structure

Stand comfortably with your weight on both feet. Imagine a vertical plane that passes from the crown of your head down through the center of your body, dividing you into right and left halves. Notice the body masses on either side of that plane. They may feel identical in terms of shape, size, and density. Or they may seem quite dissimilar.

Notice whether you seem to bear more weight on one foot than on the other. If you were standing on two bathroom scales, would one of them register more weight?

Try to even out the balance between your two feet and then notice whether that changes your perception of the disparity between the right and left halves of your body.

Now, lift one foot from the floor and balance for a moment on one leg. Then lift the other leg. Notice whether it's easier to stand on one leg than on the other.

Now imagine a second plane that passes through the center of your ears, the tips of your shoulders, the centers of your hip joints, and just in front of your ankle joints, dividing you into front and back halves. Compare your sense of the body masses in front and in back. Notice which "half" is easier for you to sense.

Nod your head up and down in a very small and very slow "yes" movement. Notice whether your head rests most comfortably at the top of that movement, at the bottom, or somewhere in the middle.

With your head now resting at a familiar, comfortable angle, notice the orientation of your chin and your eyes. If your chin is angled down, you are likely looking slightly upward with your eyes to see what's in front of you. If your chin is lifted, your eyes must gaze down a little to see what is in front.

A balanced relationship of neck and head lets your line of sight be level with the horizon. If that's not true for you, simply notice it without trying to change anything. Your Body Mandala practice will allow more balanced structure to emerge in time.

The following assessment invites you to notice a few of the myriad sensations of your aliveness.

Sensations

🔊 Practice 2 - Sensations

If you're comfortable doing so, close your eyes for this part. Otherwise, keep them open but with a soft focus.

Standing comfortably, what parts of your body are you most aware of: your head, neck, spine, pelvis, legs, feet, chest, abdomen, shoulders, arms, hands? How do you know that you're aware? Do you feel pulsation, streaming sensations, temperature, lightness or heaviness, ease or constraint, or something else?

Notice the relative intensity of your awareness in different parts of your body.

Think of your skin as an envelope that separates your body from the space outside it. Imagine the little hairs on every surface of your skin. Imagine them being touched by the air. Take time to imagine every inch of your skin: front, back, both sides, top and bottom surfaces. Notice where you find it easy and obvious to feel your skin.

Notice where you have to bring more attention to the task.

Now travel inside your skin, perceiving it as a container. Let your awareness roam through the inner chambers of your body. Notice contrasting sensations. For example, drop your awareness down inside your two calves. Notice whether one lower leg feels denser or fluffier, warmer or cooler, or more alive than the other. You might even see your legs as differently colored. Allow any impression that arises be of interest to you. When your awareness starts to fade or is replaced by another impression, let that occur.

Notice contrasting sensations in your forearms. Notice whether one forearm feels denser or fluffier, warmer or cooler, whether you feel more sensations of aliveness in one arm than the other.

Extend this process into your feet, thighs, hips, arms, and hands. Pause the audio to give yourself time to appreciate your sensations.

Now compare your experience of the two sides within your chest. Compare your experience of the two sides within your abdomen.

Be aware of your breath moving in and out of your body. Besides sensing the flow of air in your airway and lungs, notice where else in your body you can sense the movement of your breathing.

Notice whether you can feel the beating of your heart.

The next assessment is your introduction to some features of your gait. How you walk is as recognizable to others as your handwriting. Most of us take walking for granted, never thinking that it is a facet of posture, and an aspect of self-expression. Indeed, the way we walk is a moving signature.

PRACTICE

Movement

🔊 Practice 3 - Movement

Walk around, preferably out of doors where there is space to move freely. Walk in an ordinary way at your ordinary pace. Where are you most aware of your movement? Your legs, of course, are making the most obvious actions, but where else do you sense motion in your body? Pelvis, spine, shoulders?

What areas of your body seem to move freely? Not so freely?

Consider your footfalls: If your feet were imprinting the ground as you step, would the prints of one foot be more deeply embedded than the other? Do you spend more time on one foot than on the other? Does your heel strike sound louder on one side?

Notice the swing of your arms: Does one arm swing farther forward, or more energetically, than the other? If so, experiment with reversing the energetic emphasis of your arm swing. Your movement will likely feel less comfortable, less authentic, and less like you.

Can you feel your spine moving as you walk? Do you notice movement in your hips and pelvis?

At what angle do your eyes rest when you're walking? Are you gazing forward at the horizon, or down toward the ground?

What areas of your body feel pleasurable when you walk? Consider a possible relationship between your freedom of movement and the sensation of pleasure.

Add some real-time movement research. Next time you put on your pants, observe which foot lifts first. Notice whether you feel equally stable if you put the other foot into its pant leg first. Related to the weight-bearing assessment in the *Stance and Structure* section above, this little self-test has body-wide ramifications, as you'll learn in chapter 9.

The next assessment directs your attention to the shape, sensations, and movements of your body during a mundane moment of self-expression.

PRACTICE

Expression

🔊 Practice 4 - Expression

Imagine a situation in which you must do something in a hurry. Call up a sense of urgency.

Simply imagining the situation may have produced a subtle change in your alignment, in your body shape, in your interior sensations, and in your breathing. Take a few moments to notice what has occurred in your body. Pause the audio to give yourself time for this.

Now, hurry forward to meet that deadline or perform that task. Observe your alignment and shape, your internal sensations, and your comfort level.

To what degree do you feel confident as you move forward? Optimistic? Resistant? Anxious? Safe?

You've begun to see yourself in the light of your Body Mandala. Be sure to jot down what you noticed during the body reading because it's easy to forget your first impressions after your somatic awareness has become richer.

REFLECTION
A Stabilizing Habit

When I'm hurried or anxious, my left armpit squeezes in. The activity is not so big that you'd see it, but it's enough to send a flutter of tension up the left side of my neck. Though barely perceptible, I recognize it as an attempt to stabilize my body before I start to move. It's a movement error; one's neck is not a good place to find stability. In subsequent reflections I'll share more about this predisposition of my shoulder. When I was ten, Tommy showed it to me as an unconscious gesture. In my fifties, before I understood my body as I now do, it manifested as chronic neck pain that I blamed on a particular personal relationship—I saw the person as a "pain in the neck." I now regard that as erroneous as well, as a conceptualization of the sensation rather than an authentic experience of it.

What I've learned is that in order to dismantle a habitual tension, I need to fully feel it. I also need to develop alternative bodily sensations that can take its place. In the case of my shoulder habit, I need other ways to stabilize myself. These are outlined in the remainder of part 1.

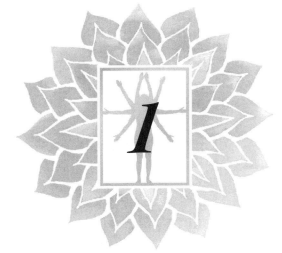

FASCIA: ORGAN OF EMBODIMENT

Ida Rolf's Organ of Structure

What most people know about **fascia** is contained in the term "plantar fasciitis." This refers to a stubbornly painful inflammation of tissues on the sole of the foot. But, in fact, there is fascia everywhere in your body. Fascia is a ubiquitous and continuous medium that contains, separates, and interconnects all of your other tissues and organs. Its significance was largely unrecognized until the early 2000s. It may well prove to be the organ of the twenty-first century.

Composed of an amorphous gel-like substance, water, and fibrous proteins, fascia is both strong and elastic. It envelops you like a translucent bodysuit just under your skin, and also penetrates deep into your body, down to the membranes that envelop your bones. It can be thin and sheet-like in some regions, puffy where it contains fat cells, or dense and thick where your structure needs reinforcing—like your lumbar spine. Its consistency varies depending upon how it is being used. It can have the tensile strength of steel wire (your ligaments), the transparency of glass (your corneas are composed of fascia), the toughness of leather (the sole of an aboriginal person's foot). Pliable like gelatin and smooth as silk, healthy fascia allows neighboring structures within your body to glide against one another. Fascia is also infinitely delicate: each of your more than 37 trillion cells is contained within a fascial membrane.

If you grasp your forearm with your other hand and move your grasping hand

22

up and down, the gliding movement you feel under your skin takes place through your loose, watery superficial fascia as it moves across deeper and more fibrous fascial layers. You can feel this anywhere on your body surface. Try sliding the fascia of your scalp with the tips of all ten fingers. (You might recognize this as the "dessert" at the end of a good massage.)

Interior sheets of fascia form compartments for your muscles and organs, and tubes for your nerves and blood vessels. These deep sheets and tubes slip and glide within you, adjusting to your body's changing shape as you move. You might picture your fascial system as a body-wide sponge—a living sea sponge, not the cellulose kind—with thousands of irregularly shaped silky pockets and tubes that contain all other types of cells. By adapting to your movement, this interior architecture allows the cells within it to change shape too. Thanks to the elasticity of your fascia, your interior volumes are constantly shape-shifting as you breathe, digest your lunch, and walk around.

Under stress, fascia becomes dehydrated, twisted, and matted, with a consistency similar to wool felt. Adjacent layers gradually become glued together, making them less able to adapt to your movement. Scar tissue is a visible example, but the splinting process takes place inside your body as well. It's a factor in chronically poor posture: fascia thickens to reinforce imbalanced structure.

By limiting fascia's ability to glide, the splinting reduces available movement in as little as six to nine months. The older you are, the briefer this time frame becomes. This is one reason that old people shuffle—their fascia has lost its glide.

We've all been taught that muscles produce movement. They do, but only in conjunction with fascia. (Fascia surrounding and otherwise associated with muscles is called **myofascia**.) The contraction of each muscle cell is transmitted from cell to cell via the fascial network and, thence, to the bones. The most efficient and graceful movement occurs when fascia glides unimpeded. When properly partnered by muscles, fascial tissue is actually stronger than muscle tissue because it stores the energy produced by muscular contraction.

The energy storage capacity of fascia is due to its *elasticity*. Elasticity involves stretching but is not the same thing as stretchiness. When something is truly elastic, it can stretch out and return to its original state without being deformed. This recoil involves the capacity to restiffen.

Kangaroos are the embodiment of fascial recoil. Their bodies are living catapults. Gazelles' bodies also contain a high percentage of elastic fibers. The amazing feats of elite sprinters and other athletes are attributable to the fact that humans, too, are well endowed with fascia.

Fifty years ago, when most anatomists regarded fascia as laboratory waste, Ida P. Rolf, Ph.D., regarded fascia as "the organ of structure." She saw it as tensioned webbing in which bones were suspended like spacers. Founder of the bodywork system known as Structural Integration, Rolf's life's work was a hands-on method for optimally balancing the body's fascial tensions. She was well ahead of her time in recognizing the importance of fascia.

> ### Defining Fascia
>
> In academic circles, there is debate about the distinction between the terms fascia and connective tissue. To keep things simple, let's assume both terms refer to your body's entire organic interior matrix. Blood, although a type of connective tissue, isn't considered to be fascia. Thomas Myers, leading fascial anatomist and author of *Anatomy Trains,* has said that fascia is everything that isn't a cell.

Paradigm Shift

In *The New Rules of Posture,* I wrote, "Connective tissue is a blanket term for all the tissues that separate, contain, and connect everything else in the body."

This sentence implies that "everything else"—bones, organs, muscles—is what matters. Although I went on to discuss the continuity and communicability of fascia, I was still adhering to the conventional view of the body.

Current fascia research suggests that we've had it backward for several millennia. This research indicates that bones, muscles, and organs—indeed, all other tissues in the body—may, in fact, be specializations within the unified medium of fascia. A primary constituent of embryonic development, fascia is the very clay of our creation. In other words, fascia is the stuff we're made of.

What if we were to reconceive our bodies *as* fascia? We know that primitive life forms emerged from the oceans onto land and into the atmosphere. We can imagine those early creatures evolving special functions: lungs to breathe, limbs to crawl and creep, teeth to tear, a tongue to suck, ears to process sound—whatever was needed to eventually become humankind. Contemporary human bodies, as specialized as our anatomy books portray them, still consist of this primary membranous material that is prior to all else. It's interesting to contemplate the possibility that our specialized organs—the reproductive, perceptual, and neuromuscular systems—might be creation's afterthoughts.

Fascia Researcher Jean-Claude Guimberteau has made an extraordinary contribution to the understanding of the fascial universe within the human body. In his work as a microsurgeon, Dr. Guimberteau was privy to highly magnified endoscopic images of living tissue. Awed by this extraordinary perspective of anatomy, he began filming what he saw in order to share it with the world. Below are two of Dr. Guimberteau's videos, used with his kind permission.

🔊 Practice 5 - Guimberteau Video

🔊 Practice 6 - Guimberteau Video

The first video shows fascia beneath the skin of the mid-forearm magnified twenty times. The horizontal white line is deep fascia covering a forearm muscle, and the yellowish bubbles are fat cells. Notice the continuity of the fibers as they expand and change direction during slight upward traction of the skin.

Lightly pinch the skin of your own forearm between your thumb and forefinger and draw it upward. Slowly release your pinch as you watch the video a second time. Picture your own glistening interior geometry.

The second video, with magnification of ten, shows what is happening as fascial structures glide across one another. You can use your own body to follow along. Place your right palm across your left forearm just below your elbow. Keeping your palm adhered to your skin, traction it slowly up toward your elbow and then draw it down toward your hand. Imagine your own microfibers changing shape the way they do in the video. That micro-anatomical dance is occurring throughout your body with every breath.

> *These microfibrils may be quite wide, with sharp edges, like knives, and with translucent surfaces, but they can also be narrow, long or short, swollen or cylindrical. Diversity is everywhere, and there is endless variety. We can see ropes, rigging, harnesses, transparent sails, and dewdrops, with rings that reinforce the solidity of some fibers like an articulated bamboo stem. Tissue continuity is total . . .*[1]
>
> FASCIA RESEARCHER JEAN-CLAUDE GUIMBERTEAU

After watching the videos, take some time to envision your entire body *as* fascia while you're moving. Move about in any way you like: stretching or rolling on the floor, practicing t'ai chi, walking, skipping, or improvising a dance. Close your eyes and imagine that translucent, glimmering, motile fabric within your body. Understand that your fascia is responding to your slightest motion, even, perhaps, to your slightest thought.

Body Perception

In addition to its role as primary container of all your cells, fascia has been discovered to contribute to your body awareness in particular ways. To fully appreciate fascia's role in body-awareness, it will help to understand three of the ways in which your brain processes physical sensations: proprioception, exteroception, and interoception.

Your awareness of the position of your hands and arms as you hold this book to read it is called **proprioception**. In Latin, *proprius* means "one's own." The word "proprioception" indicates the capacity to perceive your own body.

This sense, usually unconscious, tells you about the location of your body parts relative to one another without using your eyes. Proprioception is accomplished through sensory nerves in your muscles, tendons, joints, and layers of fascia right beneath your skin, along with input from the balancing system in your inner ears. It lets you feel the shape of your body in the space around you and tells you how much effort is needed to position yourself and to move. Your proprioceptors are processed through an area of your brain called the *somatomotor cortex.*[2]

After each of the somatic practices in this book, you're invited to notice sensations in your body as you sit, stand, or move. Doing the practice may produce a shift in your sense of the effort it takes to move, a change in the orientation of your head above your chest, a slightly different rhythm to your steps, or something else unique to you. You'll sense these phenomena *proprioceptively.*

Loss of Proprioception

A BBC documentary, *The Man Who Lost His Body,* poignantly illustrates the importance of sensing our limbs in space. The film follows the story of Ian Waterman, a man whose proprioceptive sense was destroyed by a virus. His limbs could move, but he had no control over what they did. Determined not to become, as he said, "a cabbage," he managed to teach himself to bypass the damaged nerves. Through a long process of trial and error, he learned to sit up in bed by strongly visualizing the movement ahead of time.

Today he is able to walk, but to do so, he must look at his legs and mentally plan every step. Whenever his mind wanders, even a little, he falls. None of his movements are automatic. In order for his communicative gestures to appear natural he must plan and rehearse them. Like anyone, he moves his hands to emphasize what he's saying, but unlike the rest of us, he has to spend time choreographing the gestures in advance. Imagine the strength of spirit required to live such a life as that.

When you watch the video, you will notice the puppetlike quality of Mr. Waterman's gait. For each step he must order specific muscles to contract. The movement has no connectedness, no fluidity, and no resilience. These are qualities supplied by fascia in normal walking. (The film can be seen on the topdocumentaryfilms.com website.)

Exteroception

Exteroception is a type of proprioception that pertains to reception of stimuli that originate outside of your body. The traditional five senses—vision, touch, hearing, taste, and smell—tell you about your external environment. Mr. Waterman can move thanks to his exteroceptive senses. Your own exteroception operates all day long, letting you know where you are in your environment—building your spatial orientation. You'll be engaging it throughout your Body Mandala practice.

Interoception

Rich body awareness involves **interoception,** which is your capacity to sense yourself within your body. In general, interoception tells you how you're doing on the inside. It gives you a sense of interior spaciousness and aliveness.

Interoceptive sensations include pain, tickle, hunger, thirst, sexual arousal, and pleasurable touch. Interoception also tells you about the warmth or coolness of your skin, about bloating in your stomach, bowel, or bladder, and about the comfort level of your breathing. It helps you regulate your heartbeat and blood pressure. These interoceptive visceral signals keep you attentive to your physiological state and motivate you to take care of yourself.

Sensory nerves involved in interoception are located in the **enteric nervous system**—your "gut brain." There are also interoceptive sensors in the fascial layer beneath the skin, and throughout the fascia that surrounds and penetrates all your muscles and organs. Interoceptive nerves link to a region deep with your cerebral cortex, called the **insula.** The insula gives you feedback about your physical needs and current well-being. It also plays a part in emotional processes, in empathy, and in consciousness.

Human interoception may be what generates the mind-body connection. Only primates have pathways between interoceptive nerves and the insula. It has been suggested that these pathways let us recognize ourselves, setting us apart from other mammals.[3] Through the experience of bodily self-awareness, interoception gives rise to the sense that you are in possession of your body. Because you can feel your body, you believe that it belongs to you.

The capacity to feel your body is naturally linked to an impulse to react to what you feel. Gut feelings lie along a continuum from pleasant butterflies to a sense of being bloated or to a feeling of suffocation. Such visceral sensations signal a need for response. By ignoring or overriding your interoception long-term, you risk encountering various physical and mental problems. Blocked interoception has been associated with irritable bowel syndrome, eating disorders, anxiety, depression, post-traumatic stress disorder, and even schizophrenia.

It has been estimated that for every proprioceptive nerve ending found in the body there are seven interoceptive receptors.[4] These numbers suggest that tuning into our inner landscape may be more critical to survival than is body positioning. Surely our well-being depends at least as much on being able to detect subtle changes within our tissues as it does on the spatial arrangement and coordination of our body parts. Luckily we have both capacities.

If the terms interoception and proprioception are new to you, you can make their definitions physical. Raise your hand above your head the way you did when you had a question or knew an answer in school. Your proprioception tells you where your hand is in space and how much effort it takes to hold it there. If you keep your hand up while you continue reading this paragraph, you'll feel sensations in your hand and arm such as throbbing, quivering, or tingling. This is your interoception. It's your personal experience of your arm in this position. Spend a few more moments in this posture and you may even notice subtle hints of emotion, flickering sensations linked to how you might have felt about "raising your hand" in school. You may feel such sensations in your gut, your heart, or your eyes, or notice an effect on your breathing. These micro events are interoceptive signals taking place within your fascia.

The Body Mandala practices throughout this book emphasize interoception. It is this sense that informs you of the release of subtle tension around your joints as you relax. It gives you sensations of aliveness—pulsation, streaming energy, fluidness, and a feeling of well-being. Interoception helps you to perceive the weight of your bones during the practices, and to notice any fleeting emotional feelings that may be associated with various postures or gestures.

In today's world, interoception is undervalued as a mode of knowing ourselves. We jump to negative conclusions about our interior sensations and often rush to mask body signals with food or other substances, or with distractions like social media.

Although the culture at large discounts subtle body awareness, there is growing scientific interest in the role of interoception in human life. One group of researchers has been studying relationships between interoceptive signaling, mental health, and contemplative practices such as mindfulness meditation.[5] Other research indicates that actively cultivating interoception benefits the immune system.[6] Still other studies correlate skill in interpreting interoceptive signals with capacity to cope with stressful situations and to manage chronic pain.[7] Your Body Mandala practice is your own experiential research on these topics.

Fascia is an Organ of Perception

Since *The New Rules of Posture* was published, there have been four international conferences dedicated to fascia research, the first at Harvard in 2006. Much exciting new information about this organ has come to light. The biggest news is that fascia is a *sensory* organ. It turns out that fascia—the stuff we used to liken to packing material or to cellophane wrap around muscles—actually has ten times more sensory nerve receptors than do the muscles themselves.[8] A muscle, in and of itself, is relatively insentient.

Fascia researcher Robert Schleip tells us that there are more than 100 million sensory nerve endings in the body-wide fascial network, making it your richest sensory organ.[9] Fascia is your body's largest sense organ in terms of surface area— imagine one hundred football fields of sensitivity. And this sensitivity is as acute as that of the nerve endings in your eyes.[10]

The proprioceptive nerve endings in your fascia enable you to sense your body moving: to sense the positioning of your torso and limbs in space, to sense the angles of your joints and the tension or slackness of your tissues. Working together with your exteroceptors—your vision, hearing, the balance system in your inner ears, and your tactile sense—proprioceptors within your fascia inform you about your body's positioning at every moment.

It's worth restating that there are seven times more interoceptive nerve endings in fascia than proprioceptive ones. This underscores evolution's interest in your ability to sense your body from within.

Interestingly, while there are fascial interoceptors everywhere in your body, the majority are located just beneath your skin.[11] Receiving massage or body-work stimulates these receptors and directs your awareness inwardly. This explains the meditative state you may have experienced under the hands of a good masseuse.

The outdated belief that fascia is inert tissue has engendered therapies that attempt to soften it with aggressive mechanical pressure. Such pressure can be painful enough that the effect is disembodying. Therapists who try to *communicate* with their clients' tissues rather than to break them down are working in a way that is consistent with the new research. Fascia responds to lighter touch than was previously assumed.

Standing up after a good bodywork session, you feel renewed, more in touch with your body, more in charge. You move more comfortably because the therapist's hands have helped rehydrate your fascia, and because stimulation of your intero-ceptors reawakens your sense of the connectedness and wholeness of your body. This affects your perception of yourself.

Fascia research suggests that from your outer body positioning to your sense of inner "okayness," your awareness of being "you" is communicated via your fascia.

Fascial Bodies

Human bodies are proportionally as fascia-dense as are those of kangaroos and gazelles, animals known for their ability to rebound. This suggests that our bodies are better equipped for movement than for stillness.

Fascial Conditioning

If the news about the nature of fascia keeps growing and spreading as it has done in the past ten years, we may see the fitness industry making some changes.

Isolation of muscle groups, repetitive joint actions, and training as hard as you can will begin to look rather old school. This doesn't mean that con-ventional exercises that target strength, coordination, and flexibility have no merit but rather that conditioning fascia requires an additional approach to training.

Fascia's natural endowment is to bounce. When you look at a happy kid at play, you're looking at healthy fascia. You see springiness and resilience. Another hallmark of healthy fascia is movement continuity and gracefulness. You can feel this in yourself. On certain days or in some situations, your movement feels free and easy. But if, for example, you've had the flu and have been in bed for several days, you find that when you get up to move you are stiff. That's the downside of fascia: immobility changes it chemically, making it thicken and harden. The less mobile you are, the more brick-like you become.

Similar to a sea sponge, fascia thrives when water pumps into and out of it. When you sit for long periods, when your gait is more plodding than energized, your fascia literally dries out. It stiffens along lines of use. That means that the more repetitive and restricted the choreography of your daily life, the more you reduce your capacity to adapt to unexpected movement demands, like tripping over a curb or a cat.

Poorly conditioned fascia sets you up for injuries and degeneration. Loading the hip joints in repetitive configurations, whether chair sitting or ballet dancing, stiffens fascia in a way that can cause unused portions of the joints to erode.[12]

Healthy, hydrated fascia is an essential ingredient in enduring youthfulness and elegance of movement. The stiffness we experience when we begin to age is a sign that fascial layers are dehydrated and are becoming adhered to one another. That happens with chronically poor posture in younger people as well.

The bouncy movements characteristic of healthy fascia keep it hydrated by pumping water into and out of the spongy tissues. And that's what you need to do to condition your fascia. Robert Schleip, Ph.D., one of the organizers of the Fascia Research Congresses, claims that fascia can be restored in as little as three or four fifteen-minute fascia-specific workouts per week. But you must stick with it. Your fascia will be 50 percent more resilient in six months, but it can take up to two years to fully restore it to health. There's no set routine to follow, but Schleip's research shows that fascia-healthy movement involves playfulness, refinement, expansiveness, nonrepetitive, elegant and rhythmic movements, and body aware-ness. (See chapter 14 for information about Schleip's Fascial Fitness program.)

Schleip breaks elegant coordination into three phases. The first phase is a preparatory arc in the direction opposite your intended movement. Second is movement initiated from the center of your body. The third phase is a sequential follow-through with the rest of your body. Elegance in movement is most often associated with dance, but it also correlates to efficiency. Think of a baseball pitcher's windup, throw, and follow-through, or a tennis player's perfect serve. Such actions are both efficient and elegant. What prevents such athletes from maintaining healthy fascia is that they perform the same motions over and over, degrading the involved fascial pathways and under-using other movement trajectories.

For healthy fascia, it's beneficial to seek varying ranges of movement through your joints—changing the directions of your activity. For runners that could mean sometimes running sideways or even backward. Skipping and hopping are beneficial, so long as they have an uplifting cadence. The rhythm of polka and other folkloric music inspires springy movements. Any lighthearted tune that makes your eyes twinkle can evoke a "fascial attitude." Your fascia doesn't respond to a grumpy mood.

Last, but not least, fascia responds to tiny movements, called **micromovements**, that help you tune into your interoception. The upcoming chapters offer many opportunities to practice this way of sensing and moving. So, by enhancing your sensory literacy, you help to keep your fascia in good condition. The proprioceptive and interoceptive practices in *Body Mandala* help you cultivate the whole-body expansion that makes elegant, articulate movement possible.

REFLECTION
News from Within

Yesterday's writing session was a slog. Sentences kept veering off like wayward sheep. To compensate for poor production, I stayed up late. Eyes burning from computer light, deaf to my own good advice, I was dead set on finding the quote you'll see at the end of this chapter.

Can I let go of yesterday? Of my disappointment? Of my stubborn betrayal of my body?

Heavily, I climb down the ladder (my office is in the basement), and stand at my desk, staring down at a bedlam of notes. Then, as I reach for a page slashed with yellow highlights, there's a click in my chest, as if tiny fingers have snapped inside me.

My breath catches. A flush spreads into my throat and down my arms. My chest is inexplicably light, almost transparent. It feels like joy, or gratitude. It's as if my body is saying, "keep going."

Organ of Wholeness

Your all-pervasive, versatile, and sensitive fascia is the fabric of your Body Mandala. It orders your structure, facilitates your movement, communicates your sensations and emotions, and informs your somatic presence.

In seeking embodiment, you seek a sense of yourself as a whole being—not only as a body, but mind and spirit as well. The interoceptive capacity of fascia plays a big part in your sense of wholeness. Your intuitions, your hunches, your "wild hairs" are inclinations that gestate in your body—in your fascia.

Since the time of the ancient Greeks, anatomy has been based on a mechanistic way of investigating the body. Anatomists delved into the structure and function of individual organs, trying to understand the totality. But a body isn't a mechanical assemblage of parts: it is a bio-relational whole.

By looking at how fascia interfaces with other body systems, researchers like Helene Langevin are seeking to map our wholeness. Dr. Langevin points out that the body's ubiquitous fascia is the matrix in which immune responses take place.[13] Since fascia is also entwined with the part of us that moves—muscles and bones—she's delving into the relationship between movement and immunity. Such research is bound to affect the future face of medicine and impact any discipline that involves the body.

Early Fascia Research

Ida Rolf was not the first person to recognize the importance of fascia to a healthy body. Andrew Taylor Still, the nineteenth-century physician and founder of osteopathic medicine, had this to say: "I know of no part of the body that equals the fascia as a hunting-ground. I believe that more rich golden thoughts will appear to the mind's eye as the study of the fascia is pursued than of any other division of the body."[14]

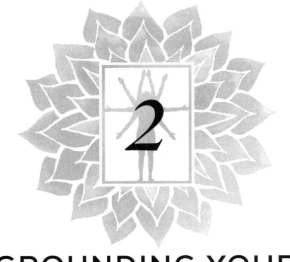

GROUNDING YOUR EXPERIENCE

Negotiating with Gravity

A premise of Godard's movement theory is that optimal postural organization occurs through the interplay of your perceptual orientation to the ground and to your spatial surroundings. This was the main theme of *The New Rules of Posture*. In the present book, I further suggest that perceptual balance between "earth and sky" supports the serene presence depicted in the center of a mandala.

Balanced orientation supports "being here now."

Our first orienting perception has to do with our bodies' relationships with gravity. It has been a popular belief that gravity tears the body down, and that's certainly the case if posture has been misaligned and maladaptive for a long time. You need only watch an elderly person walking down a city street to observe gravity's disintegrative effect on a body. But gravity can also be supportive.

Like any physical structure, your body needs adequate support. But support for physical structures is different from support for organic structures. The survival of a building depends on its stability. Once a building has been erected, its relationship with gravity is unchanging. In contrast, the survival of a biological creature depends on its ability to move. Animals and humans must negotiate with gravity during every moment of their lives. Support is a labile process rather than a solid foundation.

In Los Angeles, where I live, tall buildings are increasingly constructed on rollers so they can adapt to earthquakes. Rubber devices or springs beneath the building allow for elasticity when the earth moves. The elasticity absorbs some of the seismic energy to prevent its being transmitted into the structure and causing damage.

We, too, must adapt when the earth moves under our feet, seismically and metaphorically, physically and emotionally. Like seismically engineered buildings, our foundations are dynamic. Our "rollers" are physiological, involving complex interactions among nerves, muscles, fascia, bone, blood, lymph, and even digestive juices. Our support system also depends on perception. Our safety rests on our being able to perceive our moment-by-moment relationship to the ground. For the most part, we take this for granted.

Support requires relationship. For a cane or crutch to assist your walking, you must rest your weight into it; you must *allow* it to provide support. The prop does nothing if you only carry it along with you. For the ground—or a chair—to provide support, you must feel your body resting in contact with it. The momentum of modern life drives us to ignore the sensation of being supported. Hip joints clenched, we sit half-hovering in our chairs, ready to check off the next agenda item. Or we collapse, inert with fatigue or resistance. In neither case do we have a perception that the ground is supportive.

The experience of being supported begins within the womb and continues after birth when we rest into contact with our mother's body. The sacred and serene environment of infancy is our first conscious experience of safety and trust. In time, everyone experiences rifts in that blanket of safety. Many of us experience traumatic breaches of our trust in relationships.

Learning to trust your relationship with the ground lays a perceptual foundation for trusting yourself in all relationships. Because our brain circuits are changeable, we can rebuild our somatic experience of the safety of the ground and thereby help to heal our trust of life in general.

· · · · · · · ·

to fall,
patiently to trust our heaviness.
Even a bird has to do that
before he can fly.

RAINER MARIA RILKE,
"GRAVITY'S LAW"[1]

Yielding

To restore the perception of accepting support from the ground is, to some degree, a restoration of innocence. The practice that follows pursues this theme. My first experience of the practice, which involves simply rolling on the ground, was in a Dancemeditation workshop with Dunya Dianne McPherson. *Rolling* practice is my favorite way to recover my sense of grounded support after getting caught up in some problem or other.

Letting oneself feel supported by the ground is the primary activity of relaxation. Letting go teaches you that relaxation is not something that comes to you from outside—from a substance or a back rub. Relaxation is something you do within your body.

I like to use the word *yield* to describe this primary act of relaxation. For some people, this word recalls the sign at a traffic intersection. For me, it invokes a gradual letting go of resistance and regaining of peace and contentment. I like this word better than *surrender,* but feel free to use whatever verbal description suits you. Whatever you call it, yielding is an essential ingredient in your sensory repertoire. Cultivating it grounds your embodiment of everything that follows in this book.

To do the practice you will need a carpeted floor or yoga mat covered with several thicknesses of yoga-type blankets, and space to move.

I like to have tender music in the background when I do this. The duration of the music gives me a time frame for keeping my concentration on the process. Set aside at least twenty minutes.

PRACTICE

Rolling

🔊 Practice 7 - Rolling Audio and Video

Lie in a neutral position on your back with your knees bent and feet flat on the floor. Take a few moments to let your breathing settle and slow down. If you are comfortable doing so, close your eyes. Or have them open with a soft focus.

From there, lean your knees to the right, and let your pelvis, torso, and head follow along, rolling your body onto your right side. Let your arms come to rest wherever they are comfortable.

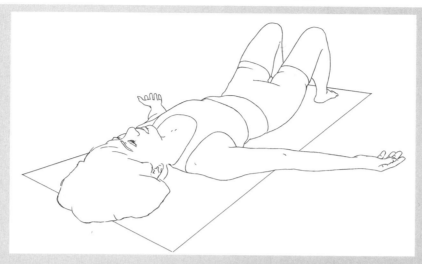

Beginning position for the Rolling practice.

To return, lean back into your hips, and let your spine return to neutral. Pause for a moment, letting the weight of your body settle more deeply each time you exhale.

Now, lean your knees to the left and let everything roll onto your left side. Your arms may fall in front of your chest or get caught behind your back. It doesn't matter where they land.

Each time you arrive at a destination, on your side or on your back, take time to feel your body yield more deeply into the ground. Imagine your body is like a snow globe. Let every snowflake settle onto the ground.

Sense the weight of your eyes in their sockets. Sense the weight of your jaw. Feel the weight of your teeth. Feel your toes and ankles. Notice all your fingers and your wrists. Sense your internal organs settling as you rest on your side. Let your heart rest. Let your intestines rest. Let your brain rest.

Imagine leaves falling from a tree, drifting down, settling onto the ground.

When you're ready to finish your practice, rest in any comfortable position. Enjoy the inflow and outflow of air as you breathe.

Next, while sustaining your sense of bodily weight, eyes still closed, push yourself up to sitting. Continue to be aware of the weight of your legs, your pelvis, your shoulder blades, and your jaw.

Gradually extend your awareness into the space around your body. Let the surface of your skin be aware that it is being touched by the air. And then let your eyes open.

Rest for a while with unfocused vision, and open, sensing attention. Linger in your sensory experience without evaluating it. Simply feel. There's no need to decide whether the feeling is pleasurable or unpleasurable. You may notice vibration, tingling, pressure, warmth, tautness, fluidness—or many other bodily sensations. Soften your focus on the words that describe your experience. Let go of any labels for your feelings. Rest in a primal state in which separation between body and mind is blurred. Sustaining this state helps you connect with your moment-by-moment sensations.

When you're ready, begin looking around at familiar objects. Sustain your internal awareness as you bring yourself into a practical state, one in which you feel capable of making a cup of tea. Practical, but subtly affected by your somatic contemplation. Practical, but not ordinary.

Before making tea, you must stand up. This feat took you many months to learn when you were small. Take that journey again now. Find your way onto hands and knees. Sense your feet and hands testing the ground, trusting the ground. Push down into the ground with your hands, and be aware of the changing configuration of your body weight as you rise onto your feet. Let yourself discover how to yield into the ground, now that you are vertical.

You can imagine your torso to be an hourglass, and you can let the sand sift down into the base of your pelvis.

You can imagine your legs are like rain sticks, and the pebbles inside are settling down into your anklebones. Your arms, too, are like rain sticks. Your elbows, and your wrists, have weight.

And you notice that your breathing has slowed way down.

At the conclusion of the *Rolling* practice, your awareness was probably somewhat internal. The pace of your breathing slowed, and it may have felt more comfortable to exhale than to inhale. This is because such deep relaxation reduces your demand for oxygen. Your mood may have become a little dull. With little interest in the outside world, your visual field might have seemed limited, and you probably had little inclination to move. Once you were upright and began moving around, it likely became easier—and more necessary—to inhale more often.

In order to move, we must perceive our surroundings. The support afforded through spatial awareness is the topic of chapters 2 and 3. For now, luxuriate in the sensations of your slug-like merger with the ground.

By clearly sensing how it feels to trust your weight to the ground, you begin to identify places in your body where you don't ordinarily do this. You uncover subtle and habitual ways in which you resist receiving the ground's support.

Notice whether you feel the weight of your thighs on the seat of your chair—whether your thighs seem as settled as if you had *rolled* into that position.

Consider the weight of your ankle as your foot rests on a gas pedal, the weight of your elbows as you type. These are regions of your body where modern life and work typically delete your perception of weight.

Every small surrender of your weight makes you incrementally more relaxed and present. Little by little you cultivate a more comfortable way to be in your body. Over time you become able to sustain the sense of being supported by the ground while you go about your practical affairs.

REFLECTION
The Ground Is Within

My habitual way to orient myself in life has been to notice what's going on around me rather than to feel my body's weight on the earth. Since being exposed to Godard's concept of balanced perceptual orientation, I've spent time teaching myself to trust the ground.

When I studied dance, I often received an instruction to "be more grounded" in my feet. But feeling the weight of my body and its relationship to the earth was not in my somatic repertoire.

Being grounded was an abstract concept. I could picture tree roots extending from my feet into the earth—a visualization often offered by movement teachers—but because I didn't perceive the ground as being supportive, the *experience* of being grounded didn't penetrate to the deeper parts of my brain where sensations and movement are coded. *Rolling*, more than any other practice, has helped me recover the perception of receiving support from the ground.

Perception Predates Language

If the *Rolling* exercise was your first experience of attending to your internal sensations, you may have found it intimidating. Sensations fluctuate in unpredictable ways and sometimes seem to mirror emotional states. At first, it can be tempting to control the transient nature of your awareness by interpreting or labeling your experiences right away. This section offers a historical perspective of human perception that may help you build tolerance for the fluctuating nature of your internal sensations.

In his beautiful book, *The Spell of the Sensuous,*[2] David Abram writes about the way language emerged out of bodily gesture. He tells us that early humans were immersed in a world in which all creation was imbued with consciousness. Human creatures felt themselves to be part of a common stream of consciousness, no more distinct or important than "wind consciousness" or "beetle consciousness." We can barely imagine what that must have been like: to be awake through every sense and to feel perceptually intimate with all of life. Were we now that perceptually attuned, the hectic pace of modern living would likely drive us insane.

Human language first emerged as spontaneous communication of feeling through vocal sounds and gestures. Most of us will admit to occasional grunts, moans, or squeals of pleasure that spontaneously emerge when we've suspended our social filters. Imagine how it might have been for our forebears, unable to contain sounds and movements of awe and gratitude on a morning when raindrops shattered months of drought.

Over millennia, the uttered sounds evolved into oral cultures. People shared their histories from voice to voice through succeeding generations. Images in the caves of Lascaux and Altamira date from this era. At that time, to look at a cave drawing was to somatically experience whatever was portrayed.

By 1500 BCE, Semitic tribes were using an alphabet similar to our own. In time these written characters caused a breach between what was perceived and what was inscribed. The characters no longer referred to the thing perceived or even to its name—to "wind," "beetle," or to "Emily." Instead, the alphabetic characters represented the movements of the mouth and tongue to form sounds. Perhaps this was the genesis of the separation of mind and body, more than a millennium prior to Descartes's famous pronouncement.

After the invention of writing, seeing, hearing, and tactile sensations were no longer participatory and multidimensional. They had become flattened onto a lifeless page. Readers could respond to the words, to the description of something, rather than directly to the thing itself. Written language split experience into categories and made it possible to think abstractly about life. Humans could now develop personal identities. They could disregard sensory experience in order to reflect about ideas and to form opinions. People began to regard themselves as separate from and superior to other creatures. One might liken this swerving of human consciousness to the ousting of Eve from the garden.

The power of reflective thought has given humanity comforts and conveniences that few of us would be willing to relinquish. Meanwhile, our capacity for somatic perception lays dormant. By reawakening that capacity we can, just maybe, withstand the digital onslaught that threatens to disembody us.

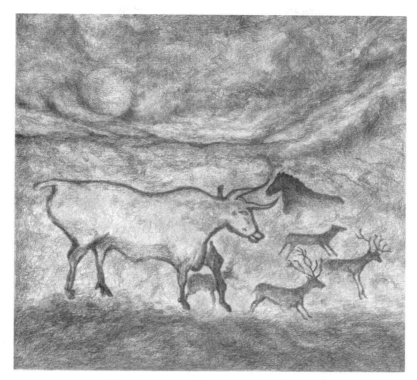

*In Paleolithic times, to look at a cave drawing was to
directly experience what was portrayed.*

By postponing the impulse to label our sensations, we give ourselves time to appreciate our experiences somatically. This brings greater depth to the experience of being grounded and to experience in general.

PRACTICE

Participatory Sensing

Take a walk where there are plenty of trees and foliage and unpaved ground. Perceive the plants as having consciousness, just as you do. Let them be as present as you are, let them breathe. Imagine the ground having consciousness. Let the ground breathe. Tune into the rhythms of the events that cross your path: the rhythm of a lizard, of a crocus or a cactus, the rhythm of a wall built of stones.

Sensing without Naming

I hope you will practice *Rolling* more than once, and that you will incorporate it into your self-care resources. Let each *Rolling* meditation be a fresh experience during which you sink deeply into the sensation of your body's weight. Rest into the understanding that you are receiving support from the ground, and that the ground is trustworthy. With each contemplative roll, you teach yourself to feel that it is safe to relax, and you deepen your somatic understanding of your relationship with gravity.

Avoid attaching labels to what you feel. Instead, pretend you exist in a time before written words were invented. Concentration on your sensory experience prevents you from forming judgments about your experience. Your body sensations will fluctuate and change according to the impulses of your being as a whole. Judgments, whether positive or negative, tend to be fixed. They block the flow of your sensations.

It can be difficult at first to distinguish between sensations and interpretations of sensations. For example, a sensation of warmth could be interpreted as cozy, embarrassed, or angry. Keep your focus on the warmth, allowing it to evolve on its own, within your body. Similarly, a pulsation could be interpreted as nervousness, excitement, or fear. Train your curiosity on the pure pulsation, rather than the *connotations* of the pulses.

Sometimes we label experiences out of a need to control outcomes. But the deeper brain regions, where your new sensory and movement patterns are being established, cannot be managed by critical thinking. There are plenty of other opportunities to use the cognitive part of your brain.

REFLECTION

Savasana

I'm resting in corpse pose at the end of a satisfying yoga class. My body is so open and relaxed that the hardwood floor feels as soft as memory foam. There's nothing to do but luxuriate in breathing. I am silky, calm, homogenous. No detail stands out, and I drift down, and down, to the fruit of Savasana—precious absence.

An odd tingle in my left palm just below my thumb disturbs my quiet. There's something familiar about it, and the moment I form that thought, my left shoulder bounces to the foreground of my consciousness. I carelessly step across the thin boundary between quiet sensing and stealthy curiosity.

My hobby, when I was nine or ten, was sewing doll clothes. I'd spread every-thing out on the living room carpet and cut and sew for hours. One day, getting up from my sewing station, I stuck the needle into the rug instead of the pin-cushion. When I returned to the floor, the thread end of the needle punctured my palm.

Now I'm off and running after my shoulder story. It must have hurt! I must have pulled my hand close to my body. This must be another layer of my body's mysterious left side tension.

Driving home from class, I glance at my left hand. There's no scar. The scar is on my right hand. I have wasted precious Savasana. And I am shown, once again, that embodied presence involves patiently yielding into my sensory experience.

The Science of Body Maps

Until ten years ago, I would not have been able to tell you why rolling on the floor can have such a profound effect on posture and movement. The burgeoning field of neuroscience has given scientific foundation to an experience I didn't know how to talk about. When we roll on the ground, fully participating in the felt sense of support, we take advantage of our brains' neural plasticity to restore our sense of safety in the world. Plasticity is the characteristic of our neural tissue that allows our brains to revise connections and create new ones based on fresh experiences.

Recent neuroscience indicates that the body is far more involved in conscious-ness than has been supposed since Descartes announced, "I think, therefore I am." That centuries-old dictum consigned the body to a supporting role in the body-mind drama, a mere conveyance for the brain. "Body nerds," like me, have resisted the belittling of somatic experience, so it's gratifying to have scientific assurance of our bodies' intelligence. Sandra Blakeslee, a popular science writer, asserts that sensations from the body are the mind's very foundation. She tells us that "mean-ing is rooted in agency (the ability to act and choose), and agency depends on embodiment."[3] To me, this suggests that meaningful living depends on conscious somatic experience.

Your brain's activity with respect to your body comprises what amounts to a mapping process. The brain's body maps give us another way to understand our body perceptions—proprioception, exteroception, and interoception—outlined in chapter 1.

Brain maps include detailed topology of every body part: feet, toes, toenails, ribs, elbows, and so on, and every millimeter of your skin surface. There are also maps for your **viscera**—the organs and the fascia within your body. So, every point inside you and every point on the surface of your body are mapped within your brain.

Your sensory maps register tactile sensation and portray your body's shape and its proximity to objects in your surroundings. These maps record degrees and combinations of touch, and monitor temperature, vibration, pressure, and infinite degrees and varieties of pleasure. They also register varieties of pain—like dull, searing, or knife-like pain, or tickling. (Surprisingly, tickling is produced by signals from nerves associated with both pain and touch.) Sensory maps of your internal organs connect to emotional feelings such as dread, disgust, shame, joy, and contentment. This means that your "gut feelings" are not just "in your head."

Your brain's spatial maps help you locate yourself in a familiar environment, enabling you to know, for example, where the bathroom light switch is in the middle of the night. Other space maps help you find your way in unfamiliar places. Still others, like a GPS, tell you which way is north, south, east, or west. Every part of your body has its own spatial atlas. And every point in the space immediately surrounding your body—called **peripersonal space**—is also mapped.

When someone stands closer to you than feels comfortable, you notice it. This sense of personal space is no figment of your imagination. As far as your brain is concerned, the space around your body *is* part of your body. When someone stands too close, he or she has literally invaded your space.

Movement maps include conscious aspects of coordinating movement, like swinging a racquet, as well as unconscious aspects, like intestinal peristalsis. Tactile and motor map combinations delineate the refined skills required to play a Beethoven piano sonata or to thread a needle. All of these maps involve intricate interactions between your proprioceptive, exteroceptive, and interoceptive nerves, as well as with the nerves that manage movement.

You also have brain circuits permeated with nerve cells called **mirror neurons** that simulate the actions of other people. When you observe someone drinking lemonade on a hot day, the same nerve cells fire in your brain, as if you were raising the glass to your own lips. And when the waitress comes your way again, you soon will be. Lemonade can be as contagious as yawning, and now we understand why. Mirroring touch and movement maps explain why we feel energized by a Tom Cruise action movie and why we feel uplifted watching athletic events or dance performances. Further, research indicates that if we have actually performed any of these activities, more of our own neurons will fire than if we have never slam-dunked a ball or hung, Cruise-like, by our fingertips from a moving airplane.

Access to Reality

Alfred Korzybski was a twentieth-century scholar and founder of a self-improvement program known as General Semantics. He posited that humanity's direct access to reality is limited by our languages—by our naming of things. "Words are not the things we are speaking about," he said, "and there is no such thing as an object in absolute isolation."

When I studied with her, Ida Rolf was fond of quoting Korzybski's most famous dictum: "The map is not the territory." To me this meant that the territory of a person's life is vastly greater than anything that can be observed in their physical appearance. Rolf wanted us to look at the bodies in our care as whole systems, neither a collection of misaligned anatomical parts, nor a compendium of complaints.

Bodies were ongoing *events* and were inseparable from their environments.

Blakeslee likens the seamless interplay of our body maps to a mandala "whose overall pattern creates your embodied, feeling self." Because body maps are plastic and changeable, your feeling self evolves not only during childhood but also throughout life. Your peripersonal space, for example, expands or shrinks to include the tools you use—a car, a skateboard, a spatula, or a scalpel. When your primary engagement is with an electronic device, your spatial map adapts to your scope of attention and becomes narrow. Confined by such limited spatial awareness, your body has little inclination to move. Freedom of movement requires that you reconfigure your spatial maps.

Neuroscience gives us new lenses through which to look at ourselves—our bodies, habits, memories, and beliefs. Our behavior is as elastic and changeable as are our brain maps.

While our maps can be disorganized after an injury, or through repetitive behavior, the brain's plasticity also allows them to be reorganized through having fresh experiences. With the *Rolling* practice, you've begun a process of revising the maps for your body's fluidity and weight—for relaxation and for your relationship with the ground.

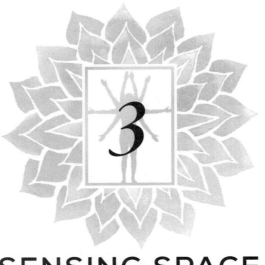

SENSING SPACE

After doing the *Rolling* practice in chapter 2, your awareness was likely gathered inside your body. Your visual field was limited, and you may have felt so rooted to the ground that you had little inclination to move. Although you may not have realized it, bringing yourself up to a sitting position required perception of the space around your body. You had to expand your sensory field enough to get yourself up. We can't move without a sense of space.

We experience the space around our bodies in two ways. We're aware of the space that can be measured as distance from here to there—we can call this "geographic space." But space also has a subjective quality, colored by our personal histories and associations and by cultural or societal contexts. For example, someone who lives in a crowded city experiences space differently than does someone from a rural community. People in Hispanic or Asian cultures experience personal space differently than Americans do.

Before making any movement, we orient our bodies in our subjective space as perceived at that moment. Each person and each situation is different, but in all events, our perception of space shapes the way we move. Practices in this chapter and the next acquaint you with your personal spatial orientation.

Simple Spatial Awareness

🔊 Practice 8 - Simple Spacial Awareness

Sitting comfortably, be aware of resting your body's weight into the chair seat. Recall, from the *Rolling* practice, the feeling that you can *receive* support from the ground. When you sit, you are yielding the weight of your body *through* the chair into the ground.

From here, turn your attention to the distances between yourself and features or objects in the room. Notice the distance between yourself and the upper right corner of the room. Imagine a line inscribed in the space between

Sit so you feel weight resting into your upper thighs, slightly forward of your "sit bones," and into your anklebones.

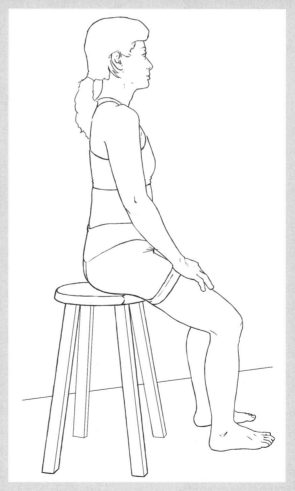

you and that corner. Then imagine a line extending to the lower left corner of the room, or to the nearest wastebasket. How far away and in what direction is your phone? Your favorite jacket? Your car? Your best friend?

And now, extend your imagination farther afield to a favorite hangout or vacation spot. Continue in this manner, picturing a nexus of trajectories between yourself and your world.

Change your position to face a different direction in the room. Notice whether this change of viewpoint alters your experience of the various directions and distances. Notice whether particular lines of direction seem more vibrant than others. Or whether some directions or distances seem less easy to access.

When you stand up, take time to see whether the experience of paying attention to space has affected the way your body feels as you walk around. Perhaps it has changed the rhythm of your steps. The effect may be barely perceptible or profoundly transformative.

Trust Your Sensations

The part of your brain that perceives sensation, the sensory cortex, is also the part of the brain that imagines sensation. At the outset of somatic study, it can be difficult to tell the difference. The good news is that it's not important to do so: in either case your sensory cortex is working to expand and remap your sensory literacy.

If you've picked up this book, it's likely you already believe there's a mutual influencing of body and mind. Because twenty-first-century mindsets are accustomed to Googling for quick answers, you may feel tempted to dive into your memories to ferret out the "truth" behind a sensation that you perceive as uncomfortable. When you do this, you are *thinking about* rather than *participating in* your experience. You are separating yourself from the present moment. The present is the only time in which change can occur.

My experience—in my personal practice and in working with private clients—is that when the meaning of a sensation is relevant to personal development, it emerges whole from the body as a spontaneous epiphany. Trusting this process and allowing it to evolve depends on being able to feel safe in the present moment. Cultivating awareness of your relationship with the ground and to the space around you helps you know where you are, and that somatic knowledge helps you feel safe.

The following meditation includes three options for exploring your peripersonal space. You will explore it front to back, side to side, and top to bottom. Pursue them on different occasions if doing all three options feels like too much at once. Twenty minutes is a good amount of time to spend. Base your practice on what feels comfortable on any given day.

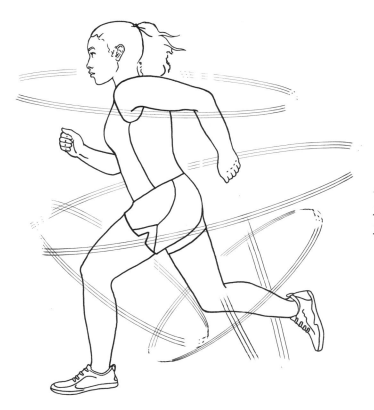

Your peripersonal space accompanies you, no matter what you're doing.

PRACTICE

Peripersonal Space Exploration

🔊 Practice 9 - Peripersonal Space Exploration

As you work with this practice, pause as needed to give yourself time to appreciate your sensations.

Stand in a way that feels comfortable. Begin to imagine your peripersonal space. Envision it as a sphere that extends from the center of your body out to the ends of your fingertips in all directions, to the extreme right and left sides of your body, to front and back, above your head, and down to the ground, and including every conceivable diagonal path.

Imagine energy streaming from your skin surface out to the periphery of your sphere.

Keep the image in the background of your awareness while you remind yourself of the weight of your bones, especially the bony knobs on either side of your ankles. Remembering your sense of weight helps keep you grounded.

And now close your eyes. Should you begin to lose your bearings with your eyes closed, it's fine to have them open with a soft focus.

Tune into the quality of the hemispheric space in front of your body: Does

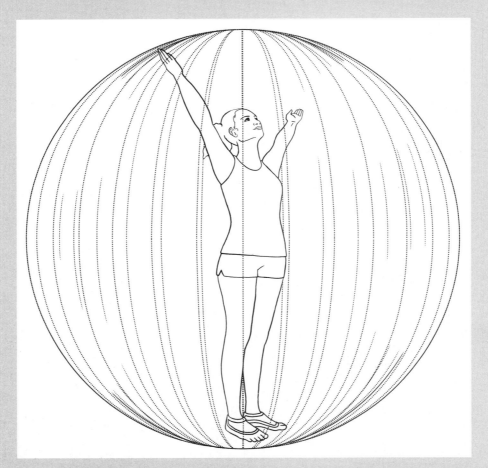

Imagine your peripersonal sphere extending out
to the ends of your fingertips in all directions.

that area seem light or dark? Warm or cool? Textured or smooth? Dense or filmy? Compare those qualities to your experience of the hemisphere behind the coronal plane of your body. What are the textures and colors of your back-space? Is this region as vivid and full as the hemisphere in front?

Revolve your body a quarter turn and recheck your impressions. This will tell you whether what you're sensing is related to the lighting in the room.

Next, compare your experience of the hemisphere on the right side of your body to that on the left. Notice differences in color, light, shade, texture, and density. Notice whether any area of your peripersonal sphere seems indented, flattened, or less than full.

Finally, compare your upper hemisphere—from your waistline to an arm's span above your head—with your lower hemisphere—from your waistline to the ground. Continue in the same vein, comparing your felt impressions.

While your purpose right now is simply to notice these phenomena of brain mapping, sometimes simply noticing causes shifts in your sensations. Be curious about any subtle ebb and flow of color, light, temperature, or bodily sensations.

When you're ready to finish, let your eyes open and take time to readjust to the ordinary world. Then, walk around for a while to observe how your peripersonal space awareness may have impacted your posture and movement.

REFLECTION
The Left Side of the Room

I do the *Peripersonal Sphere* meditation each time I teach it, and often notice a marked difference in the quality of space on the two sides of my body. The right hemisphere tends to seem full and vibrant, and when I look into my surroundings beyond my personal sphere on that side, the area seems interesting, welcoming. My left hemisphere is uniformly round, but slightly smaller, and the quality of the space beyond seems sparse, as if the air on that side is thin. Colors are incrementally less vivid. It's a neglected area of my peripersonal sphere.

A result of having pursued this practice many times is that I often find myself doing it spontaneously, in the midst of working with a client or while taking a walk. In the real world I've often noticed that in addressing groups of students, I find myself speaking predominantly to those on the right side of the room. It can feel oddly challenging to turn my gaze to the left and engage with the people there. When I do, I feel both more vulnerable and more wholly present.

It's possible that the **neglected space** on my left side bears some relationship to the retracting gesture of my left shoulder. But since both the space and the gesture have been changing, I've been letting go of my need to dot all the "i's." I trust that if there's something in my past that prevents my process toward wholeness, it will be revealed to me when and if I need to know.

Perceptual Dents

When you explored your peripersonal sphere, you may have had the impression that the perimeter wasn't perfectly round. Perhaps you found it difficult to envision the border in a particular area, or felt the edge was perforated at some point. Diminished awareness in a region of your peripersonal space could indicate that a threat may have come at you from that direction at some point in time. Remember, as far as your brain is concerned, the space immediately around your body *is* your body.

Posture or movement habits may correspond to an indentation in your peripersonal space. For example, you might lean your body away from the flattened side of your space or notice that your physical body seems smaller or more condensed on that side. It might be harder for you to make a strong gesture into the area where your peripersonal space seems dented.

Whatever you notice, resist the impulse to reach for an explanation or a story. Remember that change occurs only in present time and is generated by your sensing brain, not your thinking brain. Keep your awareness sensory rather than cognitive.

Approach your spatial anomalies patiently and kindly, in short practice sessions. One approach is to imagine transferring the sensations or images of the round or full area of your sphere to the indented area. For example, if the flat place has a dull color and the rounded area is bright, you could visualize blending the more vivid color into the dented area. Do this incrementally, slowly, and gently. Then relax and let your sensations evolve. Be aware of what you feel within your body, as well as how you perceive the space around your body. Stay grounded in your sense of bodily weight while you let your awareness meander through the sensations or movements that the perceptual dent calls forth. In time your brain's plasticity can restore the fullness of your spatial sphere, and with it, fuller capacity for expression.

The following exploration can be a shortcut to your embodiment of spatial awareness. Conveniently, it also helps relieve neck tension.

Moving from the Back of Your Head

🔊 **Practice 10 - Moving from the Back of Your Head**

Stand comfortably. Turn your head to look to your right as far as it feels comfortable. Then look to your left. Look up to the ceiling and down to the ground. Notice how it feels to move your neck.

Now, renew your awareness that the ground is supporting your body from below. Take a moment to consciously yield the weight of your ankles into the ground. Yield your pelvis, your shoulder blades, and your elbows. At the same time, be aware of the space surrounding your body.

From there, mentally divide your head into a back and a front. Everything behind your ears is "the back of your head," and everything from your ears forward is your "face." Spread your palms and fingers across the back of your head. Close your eyes and take a moment to let your head feel the contact of your hands. You're tactilely defining the back of your head.

Next, turn your head in various directions by moving the back of your head with your hands. Be very conscious as the back of your head is moving through space. Your face remains passive.

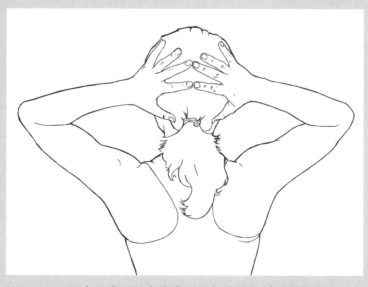

Let your hands rest lightly on the back of your head.

> Notice that when the back of your head is going to the left, your face turns to the right. When your face turns to the left, the back of your head moves to the right. When the back of your head goes down, your face tips upward. When you look down, the back of your head goes up.
>
> Now, relax your arms and continue looking around, letting the back of your head lead the action. Your face is a passenger, riding on the back of your head. Notice how your neck feels when you move your head in this manner.

You may notice that moving from the back of your head has improved the range of motion in your neck. This is because your change of awareness activates a more efficient coordination of your neck muscles. In terms of your Body Mandala, you've traveled from the sensory gate to the movement gate.

Back of the head awareness quickly activates your spatial orientation. The movement meditation practice described below helps you develop even more awareness of the space behind your body.

Walking in Nature

Our perceptions are heightened when we feel actual earth—dirt, sand, or grass—under our feet, and when the skyline is embroidered by treetops bending with the wind. At such times our relationship to the ground is tangible, and perception of our surroundings seems to lift us up. Orientation to earth and sky becomes embodied experience rather than philosophical abstraction.

Studies show that walking in nature promotes creativity and diminishes the tendency toward depression.[1] Since participating in our perceptions helps anchor us in the present moment, neither of these findings is surprising.

A Movement Meditation

Movement meditation involves closing your eyes and moving your body in improvisational ways while maintaining a specific focus of awareness. The focus in this case is the back surface of your body as it relates to your peripersonal space.

PRACTICE

Magnify Your Back-Space

The first step is to heighten your awareness of the back surface of your body. It helps to have a partner pat or rub the surface of the back of your body from crown to heels. The tactile contact can be brief and should feel pleasant to you. It needn't be a full massage. If no one is available, try rubbing up against a doorframe, like a bear scratching its back against a tree trunk.

For the next part it's helpful to have music playing, something that will inspire you to move. Then close your eyes and begin. Invite the back of your body to lead your movements. If you were on a stage, your back would be to the audience. Hold your focus on this process for twenty minutes or more.

If you're new to movement meditation, you may go through a phase when you can't think of anything new to do. If so, start with a simple arbitrary action of one arm, and repeat it over and over while sustaining your concentration on the movement of the back surface of your body. Eventually the gesture will change on its own. Your acceptance of the movement allows it to evolve, change its direction, and involve the rest of your body in surprising ways.

Allow any moments of frustration or boredom to become opportunities for expanding your sensory and movement maps. Let such moments become signals to drop deeper into unfamiliar sensations and movements. Trust that your body's actions can be generated by wisdom older and deeper than your thinking brain.

When you've finished the back-space meditation, lie down and rest for as long as that feels good. Appreciate these moments of simply dwelling in your body, the slowing of the endless thought train. Before you stand up again, remind yourself of your relationship to the ground. Take time to feel or imagine the weight of your bones.

To deepen your integrative process, take a short walk. Keep your sense of the space behind your body in the background of your awareness. As you move forward, imagine a wake forming in the air behind you. Walking outside in natural surroundings is best, but walking anywhere will help.

Notice new details about your walking signature. Do you feel more fluidness in your hips? More sentience in your feet? A freer swinging of legs and arms? More mobility in your spine as you move along? A different viewpoint for your gaze?

Awareness of your back-space helps you sense your body in three dimensions. This has the biomechanical effect of decompressing your joints and facilitating greater ease of motion. Perhaps you have begun to notice that. A feeling of ease in your body is your natural state. The body logic behind this phenomenon will become clearer in part 2.

Spacious Expression

Expression is how you communicate with the world. The expression "gate" of your mandala is the region of your work and play, of small gestures and broad actions. It is also where any new perceptual choices you've made—such as trusting the ground—can be tested for sustainability. The following suggestions help you to integrate yielding and spatial awareness into daily life.

To build new brain maps, it helps to compare and contrast your habitual and newly experienced patterns side by side. I encourage you to do this throughout this book, even when it's not specifically suggested. Here's an example of the process.

PRACTICE

Practical Integration

◀)) Practice 11 - Practical Integration

To begin, take a moment to restore the sensations of being supported by the ground and to summon awareness of the space behind your body.

Next, call up a topic that typically absorbs your mental attention. This can be a work issue, a shopping list, or a disagreement with someone.

Keep your chosen topic in your mind's eye as you walk around for a minute or two. In your background awareness, notice how your footsteps sound and how your legs feel. Notice sensations in your chest, in your hands, in your face and jaw. Notice the direction of your gaze.

Also notice what has happened to your awareness of ground and space.

Now move your body in any way that feels good. Roll your shoulders. Circle your hips. Undulate your spine. Such movements neutralize your body after the previous experience. Pause, and take a little time for this.

From here, renew the sensations of ground and space support. This time, as you walk around, sustain those sensations while you again consider your mental dilemma.

You may find your thinking process now has a bit more space in it, perhaps a bit more objectivity, or a perspective you hadn't seen before.

Anchoring New Habits

Most of us have one or two *transitional passageways* in our daily routine: the hallway that leads to the ladies' room, the ride in the elevator, the walk from parking lot to office. Those mundane transitions are opportunities to call up your newfound sensory perceptions. You can turn the location into a mental anchor that summons a new way of being in your body.

You can also secure the new habits by associating them with specific activities. Try to incorporate your back-space and the weight of your bones into your practice of yoga, or into your golf or tennis game. Call up these sensations when you do the dishes or make the bed.

How You Use Your Eyes

Being aware of the space around your body engages your peripheral vision. Having a broad visual field is essential to the perception of being supported by the ground. The contemporary workplace, where our eyes are trained on screens for many hours, skews the natural balance between peripheral and **foveal vision** (sharp, central focus responsible for details). This has a profound impact on our bodies.

Studies have shown that when we spend excessive time with our eyes in tight focus (an eight-hour day is surely excessive), the balancing mechanism of the inner ear becomes compromised.[2] No longer certain of our relationship to gravity, we are apt to feel less secure. In preparation for the fall we subliminally expect, our spines curl, our trunks compress, and our heads thrust forward. We may walk with shortened or shuffling steps. While this is the picture of an elderly person, the pattern is increasingly apparent among younger people.

The following experiment helps you notice the correlation between your sight and your body sensations.

For anyone who works at a computer, attending to how we use our eyes has become a rather urgent matter. Narrowing our focus to gaze at screens constricts and immobilizes our bodies. It constrains the way we perceive the world and how we express ourselves.

PRACTICE

Exploring Vision

🔊 Practice 12 - Exploring Vision

Choose an object on which to focus your attention. The object can be a few feet away or across the room. Let your eyes focus narrowly on it, considering every detail, as if you were going to write a critique.

Then relax your concentration. Move around a bit to restore your ordinary awareness.

Next, summon your sense of yielding to the ground. Summon your perception of the space behind your body. Let your peripheral vision come into play, noticing shapes and colors to your sides and above you. Sustaining this sense of the periphery, examine the object a second time.

Appreciate any shift in the appearance of the object or in your own bodily sensations. You may find yourself breathing more easily when looking at the object this time. Perhaps there is something different about the way you're standing—perhaps your body feels more expansive, or more settled on the ground.

You also are likely to understand the object differently. You still see it clearly, but this time you may notice how it relates to its context. Engaging your sharp central vision in partnership with your peripheral vision is a balanced way of using your eyes.

Balancing your eyes helps balance your whole body and can change your sense of relationship to the world.

REFLECTION
Baby Birds

House finches have nested in the rafters on my porch. I've set up my tripod so I can zoom through the window right up to the edge of the nest.

The father bird's red breast glistens in the sun as he flies off in search of food. Four tiny bald heads poke out from under Mama Finch and vie for the front row. Their cheeping is incredibly loud. Whenever I hear it, I step up to the camera. But no matter how stealthily I move into the room, the parents sense my presence and abandon the desperate, gaping beaks.

After several days it occurs to me that the birds sense the intensity of my focus. The next time I hear the high-pitched racket, I remember to engage my peripheral vision. I force myself to be as interested in the walls around me as I am in the nest. I move in slowly, holding fast to my awareness of the periphery, trying to spread my awareness to the horizons east and west.

Soon the father bird lands on the edge of the nest and begins feeding the hatchlings.

I assume my ancient ancestors kept a wide visual field as a matter of course, but for me, since it's a new habit, it requires concentration. By doing it I'm able to prevent my desire from lurching forward and startling the birds. There's a precious moment of egoless awareness in which I'm one with the space around me, inseparable from the walls of the room, the windows, and the rafters on the porch. The nest rests in its own separate space and I in mine. For a moment, I am in a forest. No, I *am* the forest. I am leaves and branches.

With gratitude, I press the button on my camera.

Image and Schema

Body image and body schema are terms used by many disciplines that are involved with either body, mind, or both. **Body schema** is what we're working with in this book. It's the felt experience of your body constructed by the maps in your brain. Built from the interaction of touch, vision, balance, hearing, spatial awareness, awareness of the positioning of your limbs, and of sensations inside your body, body schema is linked to the deep brain structures that manage survival. You can think of schema as an amalgamation of the "-ceptions" I wrote about in chapter 1—proprioception, interoception, and exteroception. Schema operates unconsciously, but it can be brought to consciousness. That is what happens through your Body Mandala inquiries. For example, perception of the varying qualities of your peripersonal space was a manifestation of your schema.

Body image, the more familiar term, is your largely conscious, though sometimes unconscious, *opinion* about your body. It's how you see yourself in the world, how you believe other people regard your body's attractiveness. The brain maps that create body image are linked through the parts of your brain that store personal memory, social and cultural attitudes, expectations, beliefs, and emotions. Body image can hamper your ability to enjoy life in the present tense. At its extreme, it's an enemy of presence.

There may be details in your body image that you would just as soon delete, but approaching them directly does not lead to satisfying change. For example, the common postural command to hold your shoulders back is not sustainable because it's a superficial repositioning. It has no relation to your whole being. You can't comfortably engage your arms in front of you with your shoulders glued back. Worse, this command can lead to immobilizing your shoulder blades—a difficult habit to break later on.

By becoming attuned to the dynamic sensory signals of your body schema, you begin to recalibrate your body image. You experience yourself from the inside out, rather than judging yourself from the outside in. By accepting what you feel, your feelings begin to transform on their own.

Body schema experiences are deeply somatic and preverbal. Body image develops socially and is driven by words. This is why I've suggested that you avoid interpreting your sensations and focus instead on feeling them fully. Feeling your sensations helps you connect with your schema and renders your body image more malleable.

Knowing your peripersonal space as part of your body increases your awareness that your body is three-dimensional. You feel bigger, stronger, and more whole. In a way that will become clear in chapter 7, your spatial awareness supports you.

Awareness of the space behind your body is somatic shorthand for remembering that you have the potential to move in any direction. You are free. You do not have to be mesmerized by the situation immediately before your eyes.

The back-space may also have a symbolic aspect: you might imagine it to contain the gifts you've inherited from your ancestors, as well as lessons from your own history that have given you strength.

REFLECTION
Practical Spatial Support

The first time I saw Richard we were seventeen. He stood tall and alone in front of an auditorium where high school juniors from all around Los Angeles were attending an orientation meeting for a summer exchange program in Europe. He was just standing there, shy, but I didn't know that then. I saw black curly hair, cheekbones, full lips, olive skin, and the palest of blue eyes. Did I mention that he was tall?

There followed a shipboard romance, many hours on the phone, senior proms, and college weekends away from home—including the famous one when we finally, anticlimactically, both lost our virginity.

Our paths forked, as paths do, and life ensued—marriages, divorces, children, careers. Nearly fifty years later, we had a nostalgic fling. He'd become a professor, erudite, articulate, and witty. My own way of knowing the world was physical, intuitive, sentient, and to him, illogical. How different we had each become from that randy teenaged time. Richard's passionate, Latin way of expressing his ideas now overwhelmed my Scotch-Irish sensibilities, sometimes reducing me to tears. And that, of course, only escalated the mutual confusion.

One evening, Richard was laboring to convince me that spirituality is purely a sociological development. While he mowed me down with facts, I began to feel the familiar shrinking sensation behind my eyes, the lump swelling upward into my throat, my lip quivering. Please, not again.

But this time I had enough self-possession to sink awareness into my bones and to spread antennae into the space behind me. Just as in practice, my body seemed to lengthen and fill out. I felt bigger, more expansive inside, and the space between Richard and me seemed more distinct. I found words to express my ideas and experiences without the whining defensiveness that was such an irritant to him.

We disagreed as usual, but we laughed about it, and instead of me slamming out the front door, Richard sweetly closed the one to the bedroom.

MOVING IN SPACE

Awakening: to feel our shape and proportion at all moments, with trajectories passing through us and magnetism gluing us together, all of which has been given and all of which is passing and will pass away.

DUNYA DIANNE McPHERSON, SUFI MASTER

Vectors

Sometimes, at the end of *Rolling* practice, when I've settled extra deeply into the ground, I feel like a slug. It's an interesting perceptual moment: to be alive but without inclination to move. You can probably think of moments when you've experienced a slug-like state, when your senses were muffled. Being oriented only to the ground diminishes our humanity.

For movement to occur, we must be aware of our surroundings, of a destination, and a reason for going there. Spatial awareness is the basis for our "get up and go."

When you have a goal, you move toward it along a line of action, a **vector**. In physics, a vector is a quantity that has magnitude and direction. In somatic studies, vectors describe how far and in what direction your body as a whole, or a body part, has potential to move. A vector is a pathway through space in a specific direction for a certain length of time. It can be long or short and may have a straight or curving trajectory.

Unless you're a dancer, a basketball player, or other trained mover, your preferred vectors run in the sagittal plane—straight ahead of you toward your objective. In the course of your day, you don't often step sideways or backward. To brew your morning coffee, one foot steps ahead of the other to reach the kitchen. Once there, your arms perform a repetitive set of actions—reaching out and pulling back to open a drawer, a few turns of your wrist, fingers grasping and letting go.

Track your breakfast routine tomorrow. Notice the trajectories of your limbs and torso. You most likely use your hands at mid-level—in front of your abdomen—and walk straight forward with occasional right or left turns. Your intensions and actions occur mostly in the sagittal plane. This is a limited use of your spatial perception and of your body's potential for movement.

For contrast, imagine your hunter-gatherer ancestors at breakfast time. To survive, such people must have been exquisitely attuned to every nook and cranny of their spatial environment. As they searched for game, they had to avoid becoming prey themselves. They had to know what was going on above, behind, and to their sides, as well as in front of their bodies. And they likely moved their limbs through wide-ranging trajectories to obtain their first meal of the day.

Becoming acquainted with your habitual movement vectors enhances your awareness of how fully your body occupies space. Besides projecting vectors into the world with your body as a whole, you can project vectors in various directions with different parts of your body. Dancing is an obvious example of this, with arms, legs, and spine all going in different directions at once.

You can resist a vectored movement by holding back in some region of your body. For example, your partner in a tango class might be a disagreeable person. So, although the dance style requires a sensuous closeness with the partner, the region of your spine behind your heart retracts a little, sending a vector away from contact with the other person. This interferes with your coordination, making you clumsy, and spoils your expression of the dance.

The next practice attunes you to vectors projected beyond your peripersonal sphere. You may notice that your gestures feel more familiar or more assured along some lines of direction than others. This practice is similar to *Simple Spatial Awareness* in chapter 3, but this time you will make expressive gestures rather than simply observing your surroundings. Spend twenty minutes or more with this.

Start the exercise by standing in the middle of your peripersonal space. You are always there, of course, just be sure your awareness of it is turned on. Relax into your bodily weight and appreciate the ground's support.

PRACTICE

Simple Vectors

🔊 Practice 13 - Simple Vectors

Stand in the middle of your room facing one wall. Look toward the upper right corner of the room and point to it with your right hand. Point as if you are

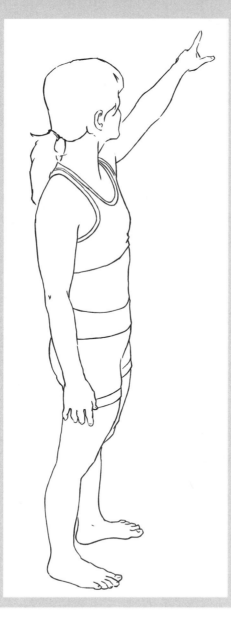

Point your finger as if you are showing something to another person.

showing it to another person, as if you are saying: "Look, see that spot up there?" Then relax.

In the same manner, point to the upper left corner of the room with your left hand. Imagine you are showing that corner to someone. And then relax. Notice variations in the energy or speed of your gestures to each side.

Point to each corner again. Observe whether you feel more comfortable pointing to the upper right or the upper left. Perhaps the movement feels smoother or stronger on one side than the other. Then relax and move your body in a comfortable way to return to a neutral state.

Now, look and point straight out to the wall on your right. And then point to the wall on your left. Do this several times to each side. Notice which gesture feels stronger, smoother, faster, more energetic. Perhaps one side seems more assured, as though you're especially certain of what you're pointing at.

Then bring yourself to neutral again.

This time, explore pointing to something at a low level—on the floor behind you to your right. And then behind you to your left. Compare how it feels to make each of these gestures.

To finish, consider which of the six vectors you just explored felt most familiar.

Your body's potential vectors are myriad, many more than six. Comparing only those six helps you notice how different your experience can be in different lines of direction. In the same way that you may have a dent in your peripersonal space, you may have preferred vectors of action and vectors that you neglect or avoid.

Like a dent in your spatial sphere, neglected vectors also influence your posture, your coordination, and your self-expression. For example, a neglected vector can be the reason your tennis serve doesn't improve despite hours of practice. Or why your roundhouse kick is strong only with your right leg. Granted, it could be that your nondominant arm or leg is weaker or less coordinated. But this is a chicken and egg situation: it could be that your lack of strength and skill is due to a missing piece in your spatial orientation. Including spatial awareness in your practice of any activity—focusing less on what your body is doing, and more on the space you're moving through—will change your performance for the better.

By working with different body parts and different destinations in space, you can devise numerous variations on this exercise. For example, pointing to the upper-right corner with your left hand will require rotating your spine and involving more of your body in the action.

You can project vectors in countless directions from any point on or within your body. In fact, you often do this without being aware of it—when you elbow your way through a crowd, for example, when you lift your sternum to extend your heart to someone, or when you tuck your tailbone under you to sit down in a chair. (See chapter 9 for a discussion of the tail-tucking habit.) In part 3, you'll see how conscious **vectoring** can improve performance of yoga, dance, or virtually any athletic pursuit.

Ideokinesis

When you imagine vectors emanating into space from different parts of your body, you are using visual imagery to generate a movement response. In the field of somatic movement education this process is known as **ideokinesis**. Teachers use sensory images—tactile, auditory, or visual suggestions—to influence the way movement is coordinated. Ideokinesis links the sensory and movement regions of your brain, and of your Body Mandala. It also sometimes sparks expressive gestures or emotions. For example, in working with simple vectors, you may notice that pointing into one direction has a subtle inner charge to it, whereas the same gesture in another direction feels emotionally neutral.

Lest you think that vectors are sterile imaginary lines, the following three variations on the *Simple Vectors* practice will help you experience their potency.

PRACTICE

Expressive Vectors

🔊 Practice 14 - Expressive Vectors

Repeat the movements of the *Simple Vectors* exploration, but this time, instead of simply pointing, reach out with your hand and arm. Reach to the upper right corner as if there were something up there that you *really* want. Imagine a thread of desire between your heart and that corner. Reach with your eyes as well as with your hand, and let your whole body lean into that vector. Then relax.

Explore the reaching gesture in the original six directions and then devise additional targets to reach for. Notice distinctions in your experience when you reach out through different vectors. Pause to give yourself time to explore this.

For the second variation, explore how it feels to push your hand along various vectors. Make a palm-out gesture, as if saying "stop." Pushing requires that you have a stable location from which to push. You have to stand your ground. Imagine you are keeping something heavy away from yourself, setting a boundary. Notice the lines of direction where it is easy or challenging to feel strong when you push something away. Pause to explore this.

The third variation involves receptivity. To make a gesture of receiving, you must be at home in yourself while at the same time reaching out into a relationship with someone or something else. You could be receiving a gift or a reprimand. Observe the vectors where receptivity feels easy or restricted.

This is Body Mandala practice: entering through one gate leads you into the next and the next—from sensation to movement to expression, or from expression to new postural stance via revived sensation—ever deeper into knowing yourself through your body.

Interior Spaces

Your torso is home to your **viscera**, your internal organs. Your organs naturally glide against one another, like sea anemones and aquatic plants adrift within the aquarium of your body.

In the next practice you'll assume a slow swaying motion that helps you tune into your inner aquarium. Because your body *is* aquatic—composed of over 70 percent water—you can sense your viscera subtly responding to your movement. Your movement along interior vectors creates shifting pressures through the fluid tissue media in which your viscera are chambered.

To prepare for this practice, lie on your back on a firm but padded surface. If your upper spine is quite curved, place a cushion or folded towel under your head. This supports your airway and will make it feel easier to breathe. If your lower back is uncomfortable, place a bolster or pillow beneath your knees. Adjust it to let your heels rest on the ground. Rest your hands wherever they are comfortable.

PRACTICE

Interoception 1.0

🔊 **Practice 15 - Interoception 1.0**

Lying comfortably on your back, spend a few moments observing the rise and fall of your breathing. Let the back of your body yield into the floor. Let the front of your body rest into the back of your body. If you are comfortable doing so, close your eyes.

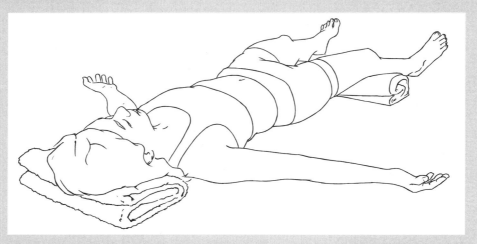

Use whatever props you need to support your body—to feel comfortable and breathe easily.

Rest a moment longer and see whether you notice your heart beating in the background of your awareness.

Imagine a diagonal path between your left sit bone and your right armpit. During your next inhalation, gently expand the distance between those two points. As you exhale, relax back to neutral. And then reverse the movement, lengthening the distance between your right sit bone and left armpit.

Continue slowly swaying your torso, alternating from side to side. Go slowly and enjoy the internal motion of your body.

Now let the slow swaying become automatic as the diagonal vectors fade into the background of your awareness.

Draw your attention deep inside your skin. Sense your organs gliding within your chest and belly as your inner "aquarium" changes shape. It doesn't matter whether you know the exact locations of your organs. It's fine simply to imagine them as sea creatures gliding and curling, rolling and drifting. Move slowly, taking plenty of time to appreciate your internal sensations.

As you concentrate on this process, you may find that some region of your body has become tense. Restore the yielding sensation to your legs, to your jaw, to the back of your skull, to your hands. Wherever you notice stiffness, you need to yield.

After swaying for a while longer, spend several minutes resting in quiet stillness. Notice your breathing. You may perceive a subtle swelling and settling of your whole body as you inhale and exhale. Perhaps your heartbeat has become more noticeable. The ability to feel your hearbeat is a feature of interoception.

When you're ready, open your eyes and move in any way that feels good. Then bring yourself to sitting and stand up. Notice how it feels to stand and to walk. Interoception is the main faculty of the sensation gate of your mandala, but as you may have begun to notice, what your body experiences in one region of your mandala quickly transfers to other areas.

Two Sentient Points

Certain points on your body are more highly represented in your sensory cortex than others. Among them are your hands and feet, lips, tongue, nipples, and genitals. All these places have special sensitivity and responsiveness. In fact, simply reading their names may have aroused sensation in your body.

Two additional points have special sentience and importance for your embodiment. One of these is located in the center of your perineum, the muscular sling that lines the diamond-shaped area known as the **pelvic floor**. Called the **perineal point** or **perineal body**, this is a fibrous fascial node formed by the interweaving and fusing of nine muscles that form the pelvic floor sling. Located between the urogenital region and the anus, it's a sensory nexus that you don't need to palpate to locate. It's right behind your vagina and in front of your anus if you are female, and just behind your scrotum if you are male. In the next practice you'll extend a vector from your perineal point.

It's not necessary to contract your pelvic floor muscles in order to move your perineal point. It's simply a location, like the tip of your nose, a place from which to project a vector.

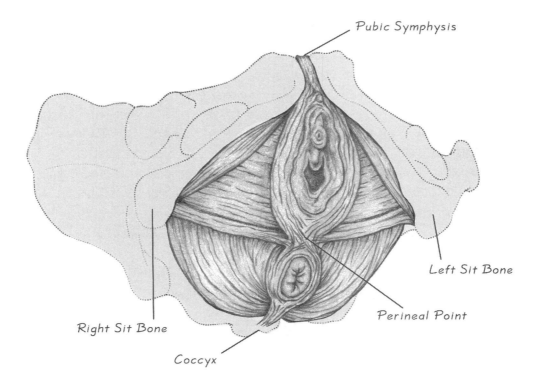

Pubic Symphysis

Left Sit Bone

Perineal Point

Right Sit Bone

Coccyx

The perineum is a muscular sling lining your pelvic floor. Your perineal point is a sensory nexus located between your urogenital region and your anus.

PRACTICE

Vectoring Your Perineal Point

🔊 Practice 16 - Vectoring Your Perineal Point

Stand comfortably and put one hand on your pubic bone and the other hand on your coccyx (tailbone). Your perineal point lies in the center of the soft tissue between these two bony landmarks. As if that spot were a laser pointer, aim it downward to make a dot of light on the ground between your feet. Let go of your hands now that you have the idea. Soften your knees a little and relax your hips.

Now draw a tiny circle between your feet with your perineal pointer. Take your time. As the imaginary dot of light moves around on the floor, notice how your pelvis tilts to different angles.

Your hips and pelvis respond to the vectored movement that you initiate from your perineal point.

Reverse the direction of your circle and make it small, no more than half an inch in diameter. Feel the subtle adjustments of your hip joints as your pelvis changes angles. Relax and return to a comfortable, neutral position.

Now draw a figure eight on the floor by moving your perineal pointer. Reverse the direction. Relax and return to a comfortable, neutral position.

Bregma

A second special point is located at the juncture of the coronal and sagittal (crosswise and lengthwise) sutures of your skull. It's called **bregma**, the Greek anatomical name for the "crown of your head." When you were a newborn, there was a diamond-shaped membranous area between your frontal and parietal bones. Called the **anterior fontanelle**, this soft area allowed your head to squeeze through the birth canal. After you were born, the soft area allowed room for your brain to grow. By age three or so, the area filled in with bone and formed the meeting place of the two sutures. It helps to settle into a quiet state of mind before trying to locate your bregma.

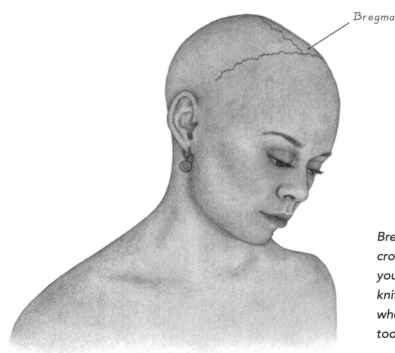

Bregma

Bregma is your crown point, where your skull sutures knitted together when you were a toddler.

Finding Bregma

🔊 **Practice 17 - Finding Bregma**

Begin by placing your thumbs in your ears and stretch your third fingers into a bridge over the top of your head. The spot where your fingers meet will be the approximate location of bregma. It is in line with or just forward of your ears.

Keep one finger on top of your head and relax your other hand. Gently probe your crown with your finger pad until you find a sensitive spot. Points nearby may also be sensitive, but if you probe patiently, you'll find one spot that stands out. You might feel it as a tiny dent, or a bump, or as pure sensitivity. For some people, merely touching that spot invites an upward vector. Bregma seems to love the sky.

Midline Polarity

Your body's midline is supported by dynamic polarity between bregma and your perineal point. In terms of perception, this polarity is the product of your orientation to the earth and sky. Your midline elongates when you are oriented both to the planet and to your spatial and social environments. Your sense of midline diminishes with the weakening of either pole. When you orient more to the ground than to space, you become heavy and sluggish. Orienting to your surroundings without being grounded makes you tense and flighty. In neither case are you fully present.

Stand up now and imagine bregma pointing upward and your perineal point directed down. It is if these two points are lodestones, magnetized in opposite directions. Feel how this ideokinetic suggestion invites more length through your torso. Remember, directing your perineal point downward does not involve pushing into your pelvic floor muscles.

The following practice helps you make use of your midline polarity while you move. In this exercise, you use the safety of the floor to combine yielding with vectoring. Do this practice when your stomach is relatively empty.

Preparation for Rolling to Sidesaddle

Lie on your back with your knees bent and feet flat on the floor. Take several moments to let your breathing slow and settle. Then review the *Rolling* practice from chapter 2 to refresh your awareness of the yielding sensation. Do several rounds, noticing that your head and torso rotate around your midline as you roll. Then pause in the center.

PRACTICE

Rolling to Sidesaddle

🔊 **Practice 18 - Rolling to Sidesaddle Audio and Video**

Begin by rolling a few times to each side. Once you feel the yielding sensation you can roll a little faster.

Now push down with your left foot as your knees lean the right, rolling faster this time. Your left hand meets the floor just as you roll across your right

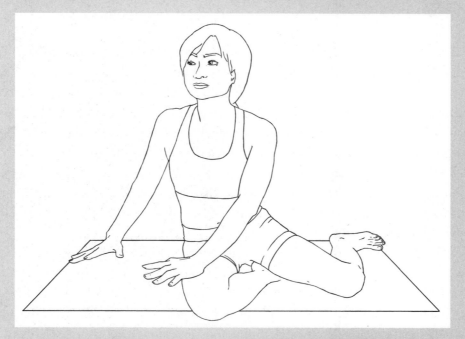

Your momentum brings you to this seated position for a moment that feels both suspended and rooted.

shoulder. Push down with both hands to thrust yourself up into a sitting position with your legs bent to the left. As your hands push the floor, picture your midline polarity: perineal point down, bregma up. You seem to bounce up without effort.

From the moment of balance at the top, let your midline fall toward the floor. Bend your elbows to ease your weight down into your hands, and let your torso roll back around onto your back.

Push with your right foot to roll up on your left side. Your foot and hands provide the impetus while your midline finds the destination. When you reach sitting you may feel as if you're momentarily suspended from the sky while still rooted in the earth.

You'll find that your breathing begins to pattern around the movement: breathing in as you swoop upward, breathing out as you descend. It's okay if that doesn't happen right away.

In time you'll find that the momentum of rolling, pushing, rising, and falling carries you from side to side without any need to push from your feet. Enjoy the momentum: you're like a weighted baby toy that topples over and bounces back up. You might even become the laughing baby.

Then come to rest on your back.

Feeling comfortable sitting sidesaddle depends on the flexibility of your hip joints. If your hips are stiff, the orientation of your torso when you roll up will be oblique rather than vertical. How upright you are is not important for this practice. The intent is to perceive the partnership between yielding and vectored movement. You are learning to feel the coordinated support of ground and space. The goal is a new coordination rather than a particular position.

For a contrasting experience, roll to sitting without awareness of yielding and vectoring. The quality of the movement will be quite different. You'll be doing it with more muscular effort and less spring. Your coordination changes depending on what you are sensing.

When you engage the polarity of your two sentient points, you automatically make use of the energy storage capacity of your elastic fascia. That's why the movement feels more resilient and springy.

The next audio helps you apply your new coordination to walking. In terms of mandala practice, this takes your ground and space awareness through the gate of coordination into the arena of new expression.

PRACTICE

Rolling to Sidesaddle and Transition to Walking

🔊 Practice 19 - Rolling to Sidesaddle and Transition to Walking

Practice a few more sets of *Rolling to Sidesaddle*, enough to feel the rhythm of your yielding, pushing, and rising up. Capture the feeling of your whole-body resilience as you rock from side to side. Enjoy it!

Then, keeping some attention on your midline, roll onto your hands and knees. At this point your midline will be parallel to the floor. Then make your way onto your feet, letting your spine unfold in a comfortable way. Throughout that transition, keep attention on the polar expansion between your perineal point and bregma. Once you're upright, your perineal point aims downward and bregma rises up. Let your feet and ankles descend. Be aware of weight in your anklebones.

Once you have your bearings, begin walking around. The rhythm of yielding, pushing, and rising can occur with every footstep. The rhythm is subtler and of shorter duration than when you were rolling on the floor, but it's there, even if, right now, you can only imagine it.

To finish, stand in place for a moment. See whether you can sense that rhythm resonating within you. It is as if your tissues continue to yield and rise even though you are standing still. This is your perceptual orientation to the ground and to the space around you. It is a subtle rhythm of your presence.

You may have noticed that getting up from the floor felt less easy and less graceful than rolling or walking. There is more work to do before addressing the challenge of getting down to and up from the ground. You'll meet up with it again in chapter 13.

Your Walking Signature

How you walk is as recognizable to others as is your face. It's a facet of your posture and an aspect of your self-expression. The idea that your walking style can change may be new to you, but in fact, it does—all the time. You walk differently when you're mulling over a dilemma than when you're hiking your favorite nature trail or entering a fine restaurant. Try on your version of those options right now to feel what I mean. Pretend you have a dilemma. Then pretend you have the afternoon off. Pretend you're dressed to the nines. Notice the variability of your expression.

For each of these frames of mind, notice your spatial perception, your relationship with the ground, the rhythm of your footfalls, and the presence or absence of resilience.

Here are a few more possibilities: walk with quiet confidence. Walk with inner resistance toward an obligation you'd rather not fulfill. Walk with happy expectation. Walk with indifference or frustration, bravado or . . . the list of possibilities is endless.

By taking time to acquaint yourself with the somatic details of your various moods, you can use them as cues to bring yourself into presence. Simply remember how it feels to be supported by the ground and aware of your spaciousness. Of course, you'll need to be willing to let go of any moods that keep you stuck on the ground or floating in the ether.

REFLECTION
Lizard Season

Springtime is lizard season in Los Angeles. Sensei brings them into the house, not as gifts the way other cats do, but as toys for himself. That cat is never particularly light on his feet, but when he's caught a lizard, he trots like a dog. During the season, I have to take the lizards away from him as often as three times a day, otherwise I'll find one nested in my slipper in the morning or find a dead one in the kitchen, swarming with ants.

Lizard rescue is best done on the spot, lest they lose their tails and escape into a closet. So, when I hear Sensei's thundering footsteps, I drop what I'm doing and get the dustpan and broom. I've tried picking them up barehanded, but they bite.

My usual approach to the interruption is to whisk the creature up and hurry it outside. My midline compresses and the path of my vectored space is a thin tunnel to the garden. I have better things to do, after all.

One day it occurred to me that the lizard *was* a gift—an opportunity to practice presence in the midst of a domestic distraction. I could pause a few seconds to feel the weight of my bones, to remember my back-space and find my midline. I could let my footsteps be resilient.

The lizard appeared to notice no difference, and Sensei's equanimity is unwavering: lizard or no lizard, he's a mellow guy. For me, the lizard moment became part of the flow of the day, rather than an extraneous, staccato event. I didn't have to recover from the distraction because I stayed whole in my body, present in my midline.

PART 2
Deepening

In the previous chapters, you have been exploring basic perceptions that help you to be present in the moment. You've begun to sense that your spatial perception helps you feel supported and changes the way you move about in and view the world. You've also understood that standing *on* the ground is a different experience than letting yourself receive support *from* the ground. This, too, may have shifted the way your body feels as you move. Together, these two resources—ground and space—are your embodied answer to the question, "Where am I?" Although you're rarely conscious of asking it, your body needs the answer to this question each time you move, even when the movement is tiny.

You have also glimpsed a central polarity within your body. You've sampled the potency of the connection between bregma and your perineal point, the way your midline supports your vertical stance and also informs your movement. And you've been introduced to the idea that your body is a sentient fascial matrix in which your various organic functions are manifest. This is a huge departure from the conventional conception of your body as an assemblage of communicating modules—muscles, bones, organs, and tubes—strung together and contained by inert connective tissue.

The three themes above—perceptual orientation, central polarity, and wholeness—are powerful resources for developing presence. But they are also deceptive in their simplicity and, as with presence itself, awareness of them can dissolve like a morning dream. Our habitual way of perceiving ourselves and the way we have been told the world works—as interconnected separate parts—dominate our daily experiences. It takes practice to perceive both ourselves and the world as whole and complete.

Chapters in this section offer ways to deepen your embodiment of ground, space, midline, and wholeness. The purpose of deepening is to become able to access your presence in the thick of things—to apply your Body Mandala experience to civilian life.

Note to Teachers

When I teach the exercises in this section, I vary the sequencing between the more active practices introduced in part 3 and the inward-looking somatic contemplations in part 2. I've put all the "Deepening" exercises in one place in the book but would not necessarily teach them in this sequence. It's important to allot time for our nervous systems to integrate the new perceptions that arise through the "Deepening" practices. To become practical, deep state learning must be accessible in the midst of ordinary life. Applying our new somatic perceptions to more vigorous activities helps build bridges between somatic contemplation and mundane awareness.

REFLECTION

Solo

Hooking my thumbs together high above my head, I reach my fingers to the ceiling and press my soles to the ground, making footprints in the carpet. Sustaining that polar tension, a delicious stretch, I angle my hands outward along a range of trajectories—to the left and right, then diagonally back to each side. My thumbs are like a searchlight that sends beams in two directions—out into space and also down through myriad threads of fascia to my ankles. I want to feel *that*, the inner connectivity. As I arc back to the right, I pass through the familiar resistance at the back of my left armpit.

On a whim, I change the cross of my thumbs, linking them right over left, counter to my original grasp.

A memory surfaces.

I stand alone in a column of light on a cavernous black stage. My solo has been selected for a concert of student works. I remember only the opening position of my dance: my left wrist is raised above my head as if suspended from a cable in the rafters. My knees are lax, and my head and torso hang to the right. With the opening bars of the soundscape, my body sways to and fro, as if dangling in a breeze.

"sometimes where almost is"—that was my title. It was the sixties, I was twenty-one, and if E. E. Cummings could compose in small caps, so could I.

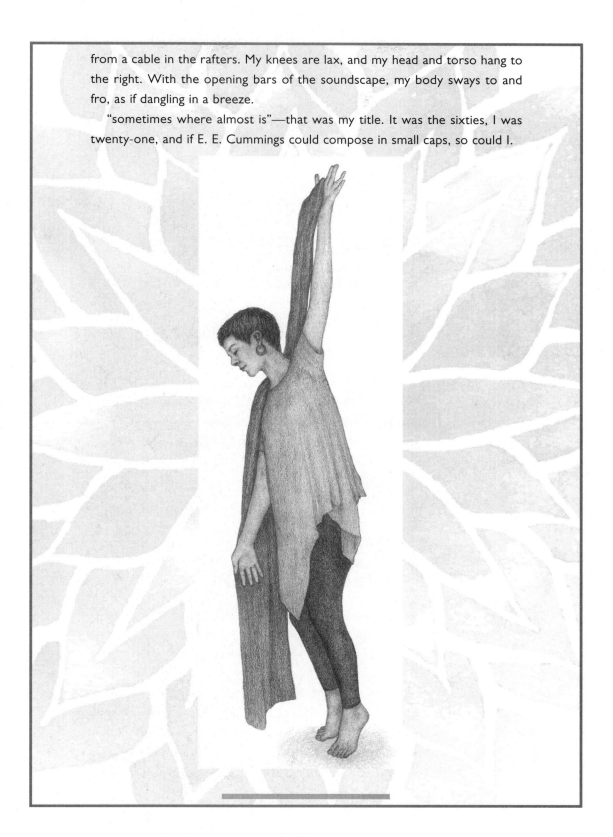

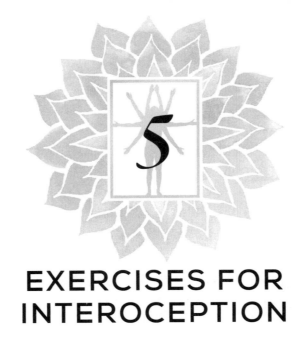

EXERCISES FOR INTEROCEPTION

It is through body awareness that we sense ourselves in relation to the other.
The more body awareness we can attain—which includes an awareness
of sensation, energy, and emotion—the more we are able to establish deep
connections to others.

LISBETH MARCHER, FOUNDER OF BODYNAMIC ANALYSIS,
A BODY-ORIENTED PSYCHOLOGY.

Interoception 2.0

In chapter 1, I mentioned that fascia responds to tiny movements that help you tune in to your interoception. Among movement teachers these are called **micromovements**. This style of moving brings awareness to places in your body that you have neglected or forgotten to perceive. Moving minimally accesses your fascia's sensory intelligence and helps restore your sense of wholeness. In addition, rhythmic pulsations like those introduced in the following two practices have been shown to increase fluid flow through fascia, allowing fascial surfaces to glide more freely.[1]

Dunya Dianne McPherson, founder of Dancemeditation introduced me to the following two oscillation practices. They've been profoundly helpful in deepening my sense of being present in my body.

All of us have historical tension patterns that have caused fascial thickening and adhesion. Sticky fascia prevents the smoothly integrated gliding of the tissues within our interior spaces. Oscillation improves the flow of fluids in our bodies and helps hydrate our tissues.

Preparation for Oscillations Practice I

Lie on your right side on a padded but firm surface—something thicker than a yoga mat. You can do this on your bed if your mattress is firm. If your neck or shoulder feels uncomfortable in this position, place a cushion under your head. If your lower back feels strained, put a cushion between your knees. It's important to feel both comfortable and supported.

Do this practice in a location where you can feel undisturbed and safe enough to relax fully and to enter a receptive mental state.

In the video I demonstrate four simple rocking movements of the pelvis and rib cage. The movements help you to differentiate the sensations of movement on the right and left sides of your body, and to notice that your body can be actively moving and passively moved at the same time. Effort and relaxation can coexist within your body. After watching the video, play the audio file, which will guide you through the meditation. Practice it for a minimum of twenty minutes. That's the time it takes for your mind to relax into a receptive state.

PRACTICE

Oscillations I: Rocking on Your Side

🔊 **Practice 20 - Oscillations I Video**
Practice 21 - Oscillations I: Rocking on Your Side

Spend several moments yielding into the ground. Sense the weight of your pelvis. Feel the weight of your left leg resting on your right leg. Feel the weight of your right leg resting on the floor. Soften your belly and let it settle to the right. Yield the weight of your chest, your shoulders, and your arms. Sense the weight of your head resting onto your right ear. Let your right eye settle into the outer corner of your right eye socket, and your left eye rest into its inner corner. Feel the flesh of your cheeks softening, and your lower jawbone resting to the right side. Let your tongue soften and fall toward your right molar teeth.

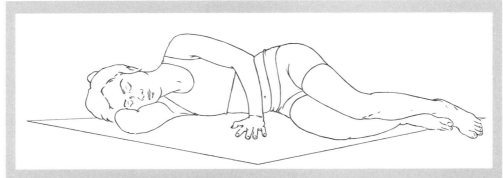

Resting position for Rocking on Your Side.

Begin a gentle rocking of your left leg and left side of your pelvis. Rock forward and back at a pace that feels easy and comfortable. Your left leg and hip shift forward and back, over and over. Your right leg is passive. Let your right leg receive the movement of your left leg.

Now your legs trade roles. Begin to rock your bottom leg—the right one—forward and back against the floor. This time, your left leg is the passenger, and it rides along on the movement of the right side.

Continue in this manner, letting your legs trade roles. One is leading, and one is following.

Now, relax your legs. Begin to rock with the left side of your rib cage and left arm. You can use your left hand to push against the floor. Relax your shoulder blade and let it follow the rocking movement. Your head can be heavy, and your neck and jaw, relaxed. Let the right side of your chest receive the impulses from the left side.

Next, initiate your rocking on the right side of your chest, tipping gently forward and back against the floor, across your right shoulder. Relax your head, and your eyes, and your tongue. You can feel the rocking of your rib cage echo upward and downward through your body, but your head and face are passive. Your legs and hips are passive.

Roll onto your back and rest for a moment of inner listening. You may feel the rocking movement echoing faintly through your inner aquarium.

Now roll onto your left side and repeat the experience. It doesn't matter whether you begin rocking on the top or bottom sides of your body. What's important is to notice the difference between the side that generates the impulses, and the side that receives them. One side gives; the other side receives.

Pause occasionally to relax your head, neck, and jaw. Your head receives impulses from the movement that is taking place below. It is the receiver rather than the director of the movement. This may be an interesting new role for your head.

Once you have completed a round of rocking, take time to return to a settled state on your back. Then find your way to standing. Find your midline polarity. Sense the weight of your ankles and lower legs. Recall your peripersonal space, especially your awareness of the space behind your body. Be aware of the weight and the aliveness of your hands.

You may wonder why I suggest spending time differentiating regions of the body through movement when what we are aiming for is a sense of wholeness. It is often necessary to differentiate things before they can become newly related and integrated in their functioning. Rocking with a high degree of attention to sensation helps you differentiate sensations within your body. It helps revise your brain's sensory and movement maps. It's like cleaning a closet—you take everything out, sweep and dust, and when you rehang your wardrobe, it's much easier to find what you want to wear. *Rocking on Your Side* is like sweeping and dusting for your fascia. It's a way to restore your body's inherent tissue glide.

Four Anatomical Landmarks

The second oscillation practice involves initiating micromovements in four specific areas of your body and using your interoception to feel the ramifications of those tiny movements throughout your body.

The four areas are your pelvic rami, your lower ribs, your upper ribs, and your atlanto-occipital joint. Even if you're familiar with these, you'll find that doing the anatomical preparation deepens your interoception. (Review pictures of these on the next several pages.)

The **rami** of your pelvis are two branches of bone that border your pelvic floor. The word *ramus* is Latin for "branch." The branches connect your sit bones and your pubic bone. We're usually unaware of the rami unless we've bruised them on a long, jouncing horseback ride. Awareness of these bones is essential for the sensation of being grounded in the pelvis and legs. In this exploration you use your tactile sense to heighten your awareness of your rami.

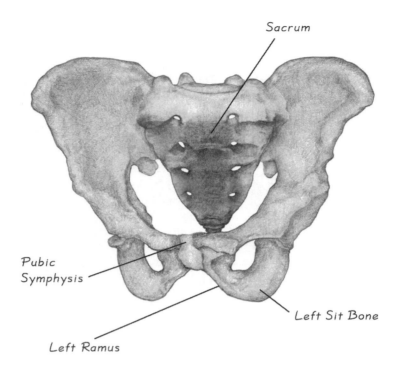

Sacrum

*Pubic
Symphysis*

Left Sit Bone

Left Ramus

The rami connect your sit bones and your pubic bone.

PRACTICE

Find Your Rami

🔊 **Practice 22 - Find Your Rami**

To locate your right ramus, stand with your knees slightly bent, as if you were beginning to sit down. Place a finger of your left hand on your pubic bone, and a finger of your right hand on your right sit bone. Slowly walk your left finger under your groin along the front of the right ramus. At the same time walk your right finger forward under the mound of your buttock muscles. The tips of your two fingers will meet in the middle of your ramus. Stay there a moment with your fingers resting along the bone. Sway your hips side to side a little, noticing how your right ramus moves toward, and away from, your right hip.

Keep your fingers in contact with your ramus, but shift your perception to become aware that your fingers are *being touched by* the bone. Let that idea slow you down as you walk your fingers back to their starting positions.

Then relax your hands and stand erect. Observe any new sensations in your hip and pelvis. You may notice a subtle change in the way your right leg and foot support you.

Repeat the palpation for your left ramus, so your stance feels balanced and grounded through both legs.

PRACTICE

Find Your Lower Ribs

🔊 Practice 23 - Find Your Lower Ribs

Stand comfortably, aware of grounding through your feet, of the space around your body, and of the polarity between bregma and your perineal point. This will be your neutral stance for any of the standing explorations that follow. Your eyes may be closed or open with a soft focus.

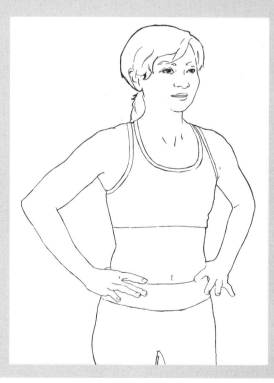

The webbing between your thumbs and forefingers embraces your lower ribs.

Now, rest the webbing between your thumbs and forefingers on either side of your waist. Your elbows will be bent and jutting straight out to the sides.

Imagine vectors extending to each side from the tips of your elbows. Then gently hug your hands into your waist and scoop the webbing upward. The edge of your forefingers will touch the lower ribs in front, and your thumbs will touch your lower ribs in back.

Rock your lower rib cage side to side. Your ribs will lean into the webbing of your right hand, and then into your left. Back and forth. The movement is so small that your elbows barely move.

The previous exploration helps you locate the lower border of your rib cage. Your respiratory diaphragm attaches inside this border of ribs.

Unnecessary tension in the thoracic aperture can tether the nerves of the arms and prevent them from gliding freely through the fascia. Whenever movement through your tissues is restricted, inflammation and pain are likely to follow. Hand or arm pain and numbness are common outcomes of tension around the upper ribs.

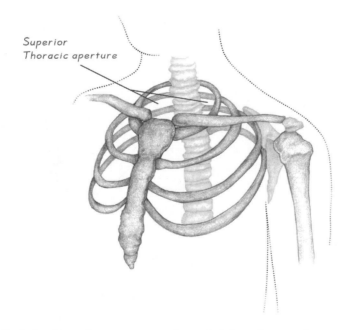

Superior Thoracic aperture

Called the thoracic aperture *or* thoracic inlet, *the area between the neck and upper ribs is a passageway for nerves that make their way from your brain down into your arms and hands.*

Tension in the thoracic aperture is often mistaken for tension in the shoulders. Learning to sense the subtle movements of your upper ribs and lungs as you breathe can help relax shoulder tension. Differentiating your sensations through micromovements helps you experience your rib cage and your shoulders as partners rather than as a unit. You'll learn more about breathing in chapter 6.

PRACTICE

Find Your Upper Ribs

🔊 Practice 24 - Find Your Upper Ribs

Cross your arms in front of your upper chest and place each palm on the opposite collarbone. The pads of your fingers rest over the tops of your shoulders. While you may not feel them, underneath your fingers are your upper two ribs. And just beneath them are the tops of your lungs.

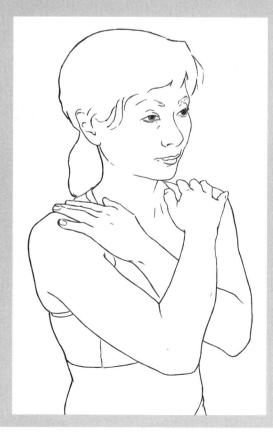

In this position your finger pads are resting above your upper two ribs.

As you breathe, sense the upward swelling of your lungs beneath your palms. Trying hard to feel this can actually block the sensation. Instead, let your hands be passive and imagine them *being touched by* your lungs as you breathe in. Because many of us carry tension in the tops of our shoulders, it may take time to sense movement in this area.

Now place your hands on your waist as you did when you found your lower ribs. You're going to rock your rib cage again, but this time, try to lead the movement from your upper two ribs. Picture those two ribs dipping side to side underneath your collarbones. The movement is tiny, with each little dip a quarter inch or less. Now relax your arms and continue this rocking experiment. With your arms at your sides, you may be able to feel the subtle rocking of your first two ribs in the creases of your armpits.

PRACTICE

Find Your Atlanto-Occipital Joint

◄)) Practice 25 - Find Your Atlanto-Occipital Joint

Sit or stand in a way that feels stable and supported. Establish your midline polarity and close your eyes.

Tip your right inner ear a quarter of an inch toward the tip of your right shoulder. The movement is tiny. Then tip your left inner ear toward your left shoulder. Tip again to the right, and then left. Continue, letting your head nod side to side in a barely noticeable bobble.

This movement is taking place at your atlanto-occipital joint—where two small protrusions on the base of your skull fit into shallow divots in your top neck vertebra. The joint is located right behind the top of your throat. Softening your throat will help your cranium yield into your first vertebra and smooth out the movement at your atlanto-occipital joint.

Relax your jaw and your eyes while you continue the micromovement of your head. Relax your inner ears, the depths of your nostrils, your tongue, and your back molar teeth. The more you can yield within your face, the more clearly you will sense mobility at the top of your neck.

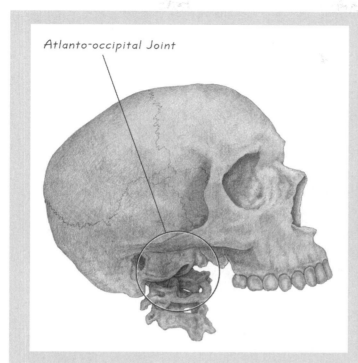

Atlanto-occipital Joint

This is your atlanto-occipital *joint—where two small protrusions on the base of your skull fit into shallow divots in your topmost neck vertebra.*

Diaphragms as Lenses

In *The New Rules of Posture* I called the above four anatomical landmarks "posture zones." The bones you've just located demarcate areas where fascial membranes are oriented roughly perpendicular to your body's midline. In the field of bodywork, these "zones" are known as *diaphragms.* In the body context, a diaphragm is an area that can close or open, like an aperture in a camera lens, or in the lens of your eye. I called them "posture zones" in the earlier book to indicate that tension in these areas compresses the body's central line, diminishing the expansive balance that is the hallmark of healthy posture.

The pelvic rami contain the pelvic floor diaphragm. The lower ribs are tethered to the respiratory diaphragm. The upper ribs lie beneath the thoracic aperture, a diaphragm-like area. The atlanto-occipital joint is fascially related to both the floor and the roof of the mouth, as well as to other diaphragm-like structures within the cranium.

In the oscillation practice that follows, you will focus on moving the bones, rather than the soft tissue of the diaphragms. As your relaxation deepens, you'll be able to feel your fascial response travel *through* the diaphragms—through the lenses—that the bones define.

REFLECTION
Scar

I'm curious to know whether an old vaccination scar has anything to do with the wincing gesture of my left arm. I've asked my Rolfing colleague, Hiroyoshi Tahata, to help me investigate. Hiro's work is exceedingly subtle. His touch is light and brief—fleeting, like the strum of a guitar in a distant room. His presence conveys the essence of safety.

He barely touches the dime-sized mark on the back of my arm. I must have been given that shot when I was one or two, more than seven decades ago.

For a beat or two, I fold down inside myself, then erupt in fury. I'm very, very young. In a flash, I remember the doctor's red hair, his pink face and glasses, and his breath on my cheek. He always wore a bow tie. I want to kick my feet and beat my arms. There are no words for this, but inwardly I hear myself screaming with bloody rage. I feel the hot impotence of my infancy.

What if caregivers knew about peripersonal space, knew that a piercing—of voice, of eye, or needle—could dent the space around and within a child's (or anyone's) body, and in so doing, affect the body's organization for a lifetime?

Standing up from the treatment table, I'm aware of an unusual expansiveness in my upper back. Instead of feeling fragile between my shoulder blades, I sense that that area of my spine can support my heart. I could now, if I wanted to, push Dr. Beaux right out the door. It's a powerful feeling.

How could such a light touch have such a transformative effect, I wonder. But then I remember that up to 90 percent of the sensory nerve endings in fascia are located right beneath the skin.

Oscillations Practice II:
Rocking Your Diaphragms

This is my favorite way to cultivate somatic presence. It offers seemingly boundless insights. Each time I practice this meditation, I take a fresh tour of my body.

The degree of somatic introspection that this practice offers will not be everyone's cup of tea. If it seems obscure to you, it's fine to skip ahead to the next section. You can come back to it another time.

Through the previous mandala explorations, you've accumulated the sensory skills you need in order to drop deeply into this practice. In the audio, I teach it as something you do lying on your back. But once you have the knack of it, it's fine to practice sitting cross-legged, sitting in a chair, or even standing up. It can be done so subtly that you can practice it while standing in line to renew your driver's license.

Lie on a firm but padded surface. Have a light covering nearby in case you feel cool as your relaxation deepens. If your upper spine is stiff or rounded in a way that makes your head fall back, place a cushion or folded towel under your head. This will support your airway and make breathing comfortable. If your lower back feels strained in this position, place a pillow behind your knees. Adjust it so your heels can touch—and feel touched by—the ground.

The video shows samples of oscillation in each area. Because it is micromovement, there's not a lot to see. The audio file leads you through the meditation to help you feel it for yourself. Use the audio a few times to get the sense of the meditation. Later you'll develop your own pacing and your own pathways through your inner spaces.

It's important to mention that there's no goal or rule about how fast your oscillations should be. Use minimal effort and aim for the feeling that your body is so relaxed that it is *being oscillated.*

PRACTICE

Oscillations II: Rocking Your Diaphragms

🔊 Practice 26 - Oscillations II Video
Practice 27 - Oscillations II: Rocking Your Diaphragms

Spend a few moments resting on your back. Observe the rise and fall of your breathing. Let the back of your body rest deeply into the floor. Sense the front of your body resting into the back of your body.

Begin to rock your pelvic rami side to side. Find the size and speed of movement that feels comfortable for you right now. Make the rocking as small as you can while still clearly feeling that your pelvis is moving.

Continuing to focus on the movement of your pelvis, now also extend your awareness into your legs, into your thighs, your calves, your ankles, your arches and toes.

As you try to sense your fascia responding, you may notice tension

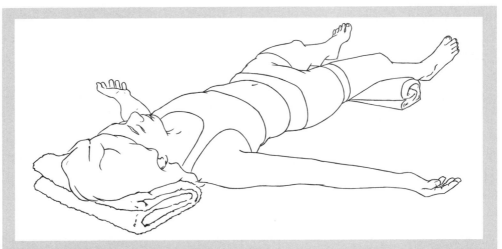

Use props as needed to be comfortable lying on your back.

gathering in your legs. In that case, it's good to pause there, rest, and renew your sense of yielding through your legs. When you resume rocking, your perception of the motion will seem more clear.

You may feel a difference in how each leg responds. Be curious about the different qualities on your two sides. One leg may seem warmer, larger, lighter, more fluid, or more spacious. Whatever disparity you notice, simply notice, and let it be that way for now.

Continuing to generate oscillation from your rami, notice whether you can feel the vibration reverberating in your lower ribs, in your upper ribs, in your atlanto-occipital joint. Continue to initiate the oscillation in your pelvis and let the other areas passively receive the impulses. You may be surprised to feel the movement playing through a distant area, but not in a neighboring one.

Now, relax your pelvis and restore your sense of yielding through your whole body.

This time, begin the rocking movement in your lower rib cage. Extend your awareness down through your pelvis and into your legs. Listen inwardly to the fascial response downward and then upward. Can you feel the oscillation of your lower rib cage reverberate in your upper rib cage? Can you feel it below the base of your skull, at the junction between your neck and your head?

The challenge is to keep your focus on the moving parts while passively receiving sensation in the nonmoving areas. It's tempting for the receiving area to begin leading the movement in an attempt to succeed at feeling something. This practice may deeply challenge your patience.

Pause again to renew your whole body yielding. Feel your upper arms resting, your lower arms, your hands, and your fingers. Then generate oscillation in the thoracic aperture. Picture your upper ribs nodding back and forth. Feel or imagine your ribs gliding on the inner surface of your shoulder blades. Notice the rib cage oscillation in your armpits. And extend your awareness down through the other diaphragms, letting them receive the motion from your thoracic aperture.

From here, let your pelvis and ribs rest in stillness while you oscillate your atlanto-occipital joint. Observe the fascial response down through your thoracic aperture, through your respiratory diaphragm, through your pelvic floor, and into your legs and feet.

Appreciate the areas where you perceive fascial resonance. Observe regions that seem inert or blocked. Extend a compassionate attitude toward these areas. Whatever tension they harbor has been accumulated by your body's attempts to feel stable and safe. Acceptance of tense areas allows them to change in time. Judgment locks them in.

When you're ready to conclude your practice, open your eyes and look around the room. Gently bring your awareness back to the "real world." Trust that what you have experienced has stimulated new mapping in your brain. There is nothing you need to remember to do or to feel.

After completing this exercise is a good time for a walk outside in nature, or to make some notes in a journal about your experience with this somatic meditation.

The experience of tissue resilience—what you feel with oscillation practice—is your fascial resonance. The elasticity of your fascia lets it reverberate, like sound waves that follow the ringing of a gong. Recall the video of fascial membranes in part 1. The next time you practice oscillating, imagine your own membranes delicately quivering.

Our bodies are fluidic, like those of sea anemones. If you touch a sea anemone at any point, the whole organism responds. The *Oscillations* practices explore this phenomenon in our more highly evolved but still essentially watery bodies.

Because we now know that fascia is an interoceptive organ, it's no longer surprising that perturbation anywhere in the body can be felt everywhere else. This means that variations upon this exercise are nearly endless. Any joint can be perceived as a diaphragm—as an aperture that can open and close. Thus any joint can become the focus of oscillatory movement.

This practice develops the ability to be simultaneously active and relaxed. The *Oscillations* practices require focusing your attention within a field of restful surrender. At any moment a too-sharp focus can make you tense up and destroy the depth of your yielding. The capacity to be both relaxed and alert is a *practical* somatic skill. For example, when you change lanes in traffic, you need to be alert but not so tense that you can't react quickly.

This exercise also interrupts the habit of holding your breath when you focus your attention on something. You cannot yield into the support of gravity while holding your breath. And you cannot fully feel your fascial resonance unless you yield.

A further benefit of this practice is a somatic understanding of the distinction between leading and following. The place in your body where you generate movement is the leader of your experience at that time. The rest of your body follows, listens, and appreciates the sensations that arise. This capacity to know when you are leading an impulse and when you are following an impulse has practical, real-world ramifications. It applies to any conversation—both conversations between you and your inner self and those you have with other people.

Upright Oscillations

When you pursue this meditation in upright positions, you immediately have more options for ways to oscillate. When you're lying down, the oscillation is confined to the side-to-side or *coronal* plane. But seated or standing, you can add oscillations in the front-to-back *sagittal* plane, or in the rotational *horizontal* plane. With more choice there is possibility for more interest and innovation but also more temptation to control rather than to follow your inner movement.

Your Wandering Nerve

Your autonomic nervous system (ANS) keeps your heart ticking, your blood flowing, digestive juices cooking, hormones regulating, breath pumping—in short, it manages your aliveness. The ANS is usually described as twofold, with sympathetic nerve branches mostly providing get-up-and-go, and the parasympathetic branches cooling things down. Working together, they maintain your inner equilibrium.

REFLECTION
Raga

I agree to go to the concert, but honestly, I'm not in the mood. Something about Beverly's enthusiasm stirs up my grumpiest introversion.

The vast space of the yoga studio is a pleasant surprise—a clean hardwood floor and high ceiling. I enjoy most music when it's played live. Maybe this will be okay.

Three musicians, seated on carpets at the front of the room, spend a long time tuning their instruments, getting the—to me, unfamiliar—timbres exactly right. Eventually one of them urges everyone to draw in close, as if we are in a temple, to absorb the music, he says.

A droning introductory section lasts more than twenty minutes and invites my head to nod onto my chest. I don't know how to appreciate this music. There's no familiar rhythm or melody for my Western ear to latch on to. For a while I watch the players as they seem to trade riffs like jazz musicians. The darkly bearded tabla player laughs out loud, and the one playing sitar tilts his head in ecstasy. This is entertaining, but it's not helping me find my own experience of the music.

After a while it occurs to me to oscillate. In fact, the vibratory sound is perfect for this. I close my eyes and begin. Time stops. The raga continues unabated for another hour, bathing my cells in vibration—soft and gentle at first—but then flickering through my body like lightning as the rhythms race faster than my ears can perceive. My whole body becomes an ear.

The applause continues for a long time. Others too have found or known ways to take in this music. It's good, now, to be making my own noise together with them, although it almost seems as if my hands are being clapped—that they are communal hands. There's a streaming sensation around my heart. As I look around, I realize that the other listeners no longer seem like a pressing crowd of strangers.

The hyper-connectivity of the Digital Age has fostered reliance on the highs of sympathetic activation. The internet pulls our attention a hundred directions at once, and as a result there is never enough time to do, see, share, and feel everything. Time pressure leaves many people uncomfortably tense in their bodies or increasingly dissociated from them. The surge in popularity of yoga, t'ai chi, and various forms of meditation, all of which boost parasympathetic activity, may be a collective attempt to put the brakes on the hyperkinetic plunging from one moment to the next.

Your **vagus nerve** (or tenth cranial nerve) is one of the most extensive neural pathways in your body. Linking your brain, heart, and gut together, the vagus nerve exits your brain stem just behind your ears and wanders (vagus means "wandering" in Latin) down into your torso and through your intestines.

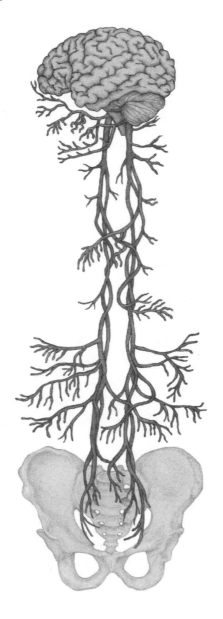

Your vagus nerve *is a major physical pathway between body and mind.*

Along the way it touches on your tongue, throat, vocal cords, lungs, heart, stomach, and the glands that produce anti-stress hormones. Research suggests it is also connected to the cervix and uterus in women.[2] Your vagus nerve mediates between the sympathetic and parasympathetic systems, affecting the functioning of all these organs.

Over 80 percent of vagus fibers are sensory, dedicated to communicating the state of your viscera upward to your brain. Together with the enteric nervous system (the network of neurons governing gastrointestinal function), the vagus nerve modulates your "gut feelings." Like the preponderance of interoceptive fibers in fascia, the abundance of sensory nerve fibers in the vagal system suggests that internal body awareness has an evolutionary purpose.

Because your brain and heart are linked by the vagus nerve, fluctuations in heart rate are commonly used to measure vagal function. Your heart beats faster each time you inhale, to move freshly oxygenated blood through your body. When you exhale, your heart rate slows down. The measurement of this variability is called *vagal tone*. High variability in your heart rate when you breathe in and out indicates that the vagus system is operating optimally—you have high vagal tone.

Stress, fatigue, and anxiety disrupt the harmony of your autonomic nervous system by over-activating the sympathetic branch. This irritates the vagus nerve, leading to many gastric, heart, and respiratory symptoms, degrading the immune system, and causing inflammation.

Poor posture can also cause the vagus to misfire. A curled, compressed posture of the torso and spine is associated with sympathetic activation. The parasympathetic nervous system is active when your throat, heart, and belly are comfortably open and exposed—that is, when your midline polarity is fully extended—and when breathing is unimpeded.

When all is well, your vagus nerve contributes to your somatic presence in vital ways. Through its connection to the organs of expression in your face and throat and to your middle ear muscles, the vagus nerve helps you be present in your interactions with other people. High vagal tone increases your capacity for communication, empathy, and friendship. Such positive social connection is a proven factor in general health. Low vagal tone is linked to inflammation, negative moods, loneliness, and heart attacks.

Bodywork that releases the myofascia has been shown to increase vagal tone. It stands to reason—though it has not yet been studied—that fascia-targeted exercise, as described in chapter 1, would also contribute to high vagal tone. Such exercise includes rhythmic movements that recruit fascia's elastic capacity, movements that are nonrepetitive and novel, movements that engage the body as a whole, and micromovements that stimulate interoception. Such movement tunes your body, in the same way that you tune a stringed instrument in order to produce a harmonious and pleasing sound. It would be interesting to measure your vagal tone after a deep round of *Oscillations* practice.*

Emotions associated with high vagal tone are trust, love, compassion, and acceptance. Behavioral neuroscientist Stephen Porges, who has been researching and writing about the vagus nerve for many years, sees its optimal functioning as essential to human survival. He points out that "the embodied experience is critical to humans because being interactive with others is critical for human survival."[3]

To be embodied involves being able to recognize your body's interoceptive signals. You notice the bodily sensations associated with what you're doing, where you're located, and whom you're with. Rather than overriding or ignoring uncomfortable sensations, you value them enough to seek comfortable circumstances whenever you can. Respecting your body's signals is a way of tending to your vagal tone. In respecting your own comfort, you learn to respect others' needs as well.[4]

REFLECTION
Raga Reverberation

When I left the raga concert, I felt more generous toward my fellow humans than I had before the evening began. Was this due to the trance-inducing nature of the music? Was it caused by my deepening interoception? By the slowing of my breathing? I'm pretty sure my vagus nerve had something to do with it.

Challenges of Inner Travel

Bodily sensations are ever-changing and unpredictable, so going inside to feel them involves a degree of risk. When you enter a deep state within yourself, sensation in parts of your body that you have not been aware of may unexpectedly surface.

Most of us have experienced some degree of traumatic stress in our lives, times when we have been in an unsafe situation or have felt threatened. At such times our nervous system activates any of three modes of defense. "Fight" and "flight" in

---

*The Feldenkrais Method and Continuum Movement are two other somatic practices that invite deep attention to sensorimotor details.

the "fight or flight" defense are commonly understood survival tactics.

But there's a third mode of defense—immobilization or "freeze." This archaic, reptilian form of survival is mediated by the vagal system.

When we've shut down in response to something fearful, it's common to lose relationship to all or part of the body, even though the threat has passed. We can remain dissociated for a long time. Healing—becoming whole—involves reintegrating awareness of neglected areas of the body.

Somatic awareness practices such as *Rolling, Spatial Awareness,* and *Oscillations* have the potential to facilitate reintegration. In doing so, they may draw forth forgotten sensations. This is why it's important to be in a safe and undisturbed location when you practice the somatic contemplations in this book or any other type of meditation.

Should you find yourself feeling anxious as your practice deepens, slow down. Practice in short stages of less than fifteen minutes. You'll gradually build up a tolerance for your internal sensations, but that can't happen if you push yourself over the border of what feels comfortable on any given day.

As recommended in chapter 2, keep your focus on the sensations themselves—the physical feelings—rather than trying to discern their meaning. Staying present with your sensations allows them to be reinterpreted by your body schema and remapped by your brain. Labeling your sensations turns them into cognitive experience and sabotages your embodiment.

Tracking Vagal Tone through Your Body Mandala

It would seem that anything that cultivates high vagal tone also supports development of our best selves and contributes to the somatic presence we are seeking.

When you activate the vector between bregma and your perineal point, you engage deep back extensor muscles, the ones that support your upright posture. This is a powerful stance because it makes your body bigger. It's also a vulnerable stance because it exposes your internal organs. Through repeated exposure—and thanks to your brain's plasticity—expansive posture can gradually become comfortable. Open posture gives the vagus nerve more space in which to function. Since high vagal tone is correlated with feeling safe, this is a win-win situation.

Practicing the physical sensations that support being fully present also helps you to feel safe. Feeling—again and again—the sensation of being supported by the ground teaches you to recognize the sensations of safety. It maps your brain with the potential to feel safe in any moment. This leads to practical and expressive actions: feeling safe helps us feel big enough to engage with the world in new ways.

Studies have shown that disciplines such as *mindfulness* and *loving-kindness meditation* practices have helped participants raise vagal tone. By cultivating interoception and body awareness in general, our bodies become the focus of meditative moments throughout the day. No one has yet done a study about the effect of recurrent short moments of equanimity and presence. Perhaps you have a gut feeling about the potential results of such a study.

Diaphragmatic breathing with extended exhalation practiced in pranayama yoga has been correlated to high vagal tone. Chronic hyperventilation—poor breathing habits—cause the same maladies as low vagal tone. Thus, it's logical to assume that healthy breathing habits in general would elevate vagal tone. Breath awareness is the focus of chapter 6.

What would life be like if creative people felt safe, or more people could become creative because they felt safe?

STEPHEN PORGES

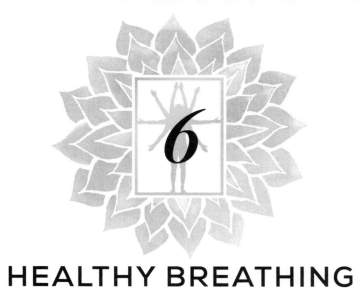

HEALTHY BREATHING

How you breathe makes a big difference in the quality of your life. **Pranayama**, a yogic breathing discipline, has been shown to raise vagal tone and reduce the production of stress hormones in the body. While outside the scope of this book, pranayama practice could be a beneficial addition to your personal Body Mandala journey.

My intent is to help you cultivate healthy breathing during daily life, so that even without practicing pranayama, you can feel calmer, more centered, and more positive. The practices in this chapter are intended to help you understand your breathing as a whole-body phenomenon, rather than to learn a specific breathing practice.

A Brief Tour of Breathing Anatomy

Your diaphragm is a thin, dome-shaped expanse of muscle that forms a boundary between the organs of your rib cage and the organs of your abdomen. Drawings of the diaphragm in anatomy books make it look more substantial than it is. It's quite thin, like a slice of prosciutto between slippery layers of fascial membrane. When you inhale, your diaphragm contracts in a way that flattens it downward toward your belly, pushing your belly out a little bit. When you exhale, it relaxes back into the dome shape. The dome of your diaphragm descends one or two centimeters when you're relaxed but can move up to ten centimeters during exercise.

There's no single right way to breathe. The amount of oxygen you need depends on how active you are. When you're lying down, resting quietly, the diaphragm's

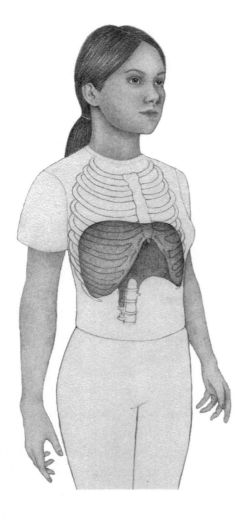

Your diaphragm flattens down when you inhale and relaxes back up to its dome shape when you exhale.

contractions draw in all the air you need. It works like this: your lungs are attached to a membranous lining on the inner surface of your rib cage and to the top of your diaphragm. When your diaphragm contracts and descends, it causes your rib cage to expand, stretching the attached lung tissue. The resulting expansion of the inner space within your lungs creates a vacuum that nature wants to fill—air rushes in. When your diaphragm relaxes, air flows out.

When you're seated or standing, you need more oxygen than you do when you're lying down because being upright requires more energy. Inhaling more deeply recruits accessory breathing muscles that further expand your rib cage. These muscles rotate your individual ribs, tipping them up and down like venetian blinds. In order for the ribs to rotate at their junctures with the vertebrae, the spine lengthens, and the vertebrae minutely separate. If you're moving vigorously, your accessory inhalation muscles work even harder. With strenuous activity you also recruit abdominal muscles to help you exhale the increased volume of air.

Respiration is most efficient when you breathe through your nose. Infants must breathe through their noses in order to suckle, and we're all born knowing how. For various reasons, a person may develop a habit of mouth breathing and will need to relearn to breathe with the nose.

Nasal breathing stimulates contraction of the diaphragm, drawing air into the lower lungs. The lower lungs are dense with capillaries, the tiny blood vessels where oxygen and carbon dioxide are exchanged. Mouth breathing tends to activate only the upper rib cage and upper lungs where there are fewer capillaries. It's good that we can use the mouth for emergency breathing if something has immobilized the diaphragm—a blow to the abdomen, for example. But because it's connected with emergencies, mouth breathing keys us into the sympathetic nervous system. Sympathetic activation lowers vagal tone.

Up to 30 percent of people suffer from a condition known as **chronic hyperventilation syndrome**. This results from breathing too shallowly and too fast, combined with the periodic overreaction of taking in too much air at once. People with this syndrome sigh and yawn a great deal and are often mouth breathers. In time this breathing dysfunction alters normal body chemistry, upsetting the chemical balance between oxygen and carbon dioxide in the blood. This leads to a variety of seemingly unrelated symptoms such as erratic blood pressure, upset stomach, bloated sensations, sexual problems, achy muscles, depression, and anxiety. Recall that many of these dysfunctions have also been associated with disrupted interoception.

The combined actions of your ribs, spine, and diaphragm result in a three-dimensional motion of the rib cage. When this full breathing response is inhibited by illness, trauma or prolonged mundane stress, the result is dysfunctional breathing habits. One of these habits is to block the diaphragm's descent with abdominal tension. This results in a pattern of shallow, upper-chest breathing. Another habit is failure to expand the breath into the back of the rib cage where the bulk of lung tissue is located. Breath awareness in yoga's Child's pose is a way to begin revising these two habits.*

---

*For a more thorough discussion of the physiology of breathing and of the surprising symptoms caused by poor breathing habits, please refer to chapter 4 of *The New Rules of Posture*.

Fascial Resonance and Breath

In the breathing section of my first book, I used the term "fascial breathing" for an exercise in which I invited readers to sense the body-wide movement of breathing. This was in 1991, before scientific researchers had revealed the sensory capacity of fascia. Early readers of *Balancing Your Body* had to take it on faith that respiration, occurring in the lungs, could be perceived anywhere and everywhere in the body. Today our capacity to feel such things is scientifically affirmed.

PRACTICE

Breathing in Child's Pose

🔊 **Practice 28 - Breathing in Child Pose**

Kneel on a firm but padded surface. Have your big toes touching and your knees apart. Let your sit bones rest onto your heels.

If your ankles feel stiff in this position, place a small, rolled towel beneath them for support. If the position stresses your knees, place a folded towel

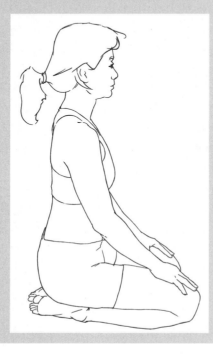

Kneeling with your sit bones resting onto your heels.

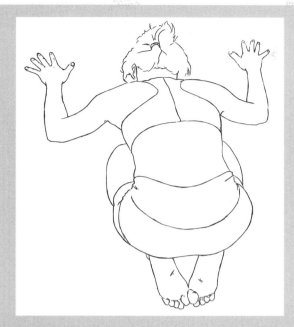

Resting in Child's pose with a long midline and ample space for your internal organs.

between your calves and the backs of your thighs. If your sit bones don't comfortably reach your heels, use a cushion to fill in the gap. It's important to be comfortable so that you can yield. Have a folded towel or book nearby. You'll use it as a prop under your forehead when you settle into Child's pose.

Be aware of the weight of your body resting onto your shins and heels, or into the chair if you are seated. Recall the polarity between bregma and your perineal point. Breathe gently.

Picture the front of your spine within your torso. It is about a third of the way forward from the surface of your back and just behind your internal organs.

Continuing to breathe easily, picture your bladder in front of your sacrum. Imagine your intestines in front of your lower spine. Your stomach and your diaphragm lie in front of your middle spine. Your heart and lungs are in front of your upper spine. And your airway and esophagus are in front of your neck vertebrae. Your organs are the sea creatures in your internal aquarium. They move around a little in response to the rise and fall of your breathing. Take a moment to sense that.

To move into Child's pose, first lean forward from your hip joints, and then let your head and spine round gently forward. Your midline remains long as it curves forward and down. As your spine settles into Child's pose, it stays elongated, leaving plenty of room for your internal organs.

Rest your forehead onto your prop. Spread your palms out on the ground beside your head. Have your elbows bent and yield the weight of your arms and hands to the ground. Imagine vectors emanating out to each side from the tips of your elbows.

Let the weight of your forehead rest deeply into the prop. Perceive the weight of your lower jawbone, your lips, and your teeth. Feel the weight of your pelvis resting on your legs.

Feel your tongue resting lightly against the roof of your mouth. Let your tongue widen and gently spread out toward the inside surfaces of your upper molar teeth. Breathe in and out through your nose.

As you inhale, your diaphragm descends toward your belly, and you can feel your belly swell against your thighs. As you exhale your belly recedes into your abdominal cavity. Simply observe this activity without forcing it to happen. Each time you exhale, let your shins and forehead sink more deeply and restfully into the ground.

Now become aware of the movement of your breathing in your lower back rib cage. This is where your lungs have the most capillaries available for oxygen exchange. Imagine the venetian blinds on either side of your spine tilting upward as you breathe in and downward as you breathe out.

With your inhalation inflating the back of your rib cage, you may notice that your elbows seem to glide apart from one another, and your collarbones glide away from your breastbone. Your inhalation makes room inside your body. It lengthens the back of your spine and the front of your spine.

Exhalation lets the tissues in your body settle without making you feel smaller.

To finish, push yourself onto hands and knees. Extend one leg at a time to stretch out your knees and hips.

Before standing up, spend several moments in an upright kneeling position. Look for the sensation of your back rib cage swelling with your inhalation. Picture the front of your spine lengthening at the same time that your lower back rib cage fills. When you exhale, yield your body's weight into the ground. Appreciate the way the earth supports your body.

Once you are standing up again, ask yourself the mandala questions: What do you sense in your body as a result of this breathing practice? Has it impacted your stance? The way you see the world around you? How your movement feels as you walk around?

Fascial breathing is quite striking the first time you tune into it. It might even seem "freaky" if you're not used to being intimate with your own aliveness. Fascial breathing lets you know you're alive in your body. This may touch your vulnerability, reminding you of your impermanence.

Each of your vertebrae rests within your fascial matrix. Your ligaments, tendons, and **spinal discs** are all types of fascia. In normal inhalation the fascia stretches a tiny bit so the vertebrae can spread minutely apart from each other. This decompresses the spine. The next time you breathe in Child's pose, observe where along your spine you actually feel that movement. Most people will notice a few spinal segments that don't respond to the breath movement. In chapters 9 through 11, you will experience options for changing the brain mapping of immovable vertebrae. For now, simply observe them.

REFLECTION
Stopping Time

I'm late. If I miss this appointment with Myrna, I'll have to wait another six weeks. Nobody ever cancels.

There's a bottleneck on Silver Lake Boulevard where it curves around past the dog park. Please, *please, move on!* My hand hovers over the horn.

My foot is poised to clap on the brake. My ankle is carved from stone. My sit bones draw up from the seat, my chest hunkers into my solar plexus, and my left shoulder ticks inward a notch. I'm the opposite of expanded. I'm barely breathing.

It's not effective, this effort to stop time. For that's what I'm trying to do. It's a crazy bargain: if I don't breathe, then I'm not living, and therefore time is not passing. But time *is* passing for Myrna. Holding *my* breath has no effect on Myrna's time.

Traffic inches along beside the vast concrete emptiness of Silver Lake. The beautiful reservoir has been temporarily drained because it no longer meets federal drinking water standards. People are worried about pollution, terrorism, and natural disasters. And I'm worrying about a haircut. I might as well unclench my buttocks, unkink my spine, and gaze at the happy dogs sniffing one another on a pleasantly cool Los Angeles day.

I'm grateful to be able to so quickly interrupt my attempt to stop time. Learning to do this took years of attention and practice, and, at some point, a deep inner decision to be done with that particular habit.

Restful Breathing

Along with rib cage expansion and spine **extension**, breathing motions also occur in your arms and face. The next meditation invites you to sense these normal motions. The first time you listen to the *Restful Breathing* audio, you may find there are too many details to take in. It's fine to pause the audio to divide this meditation into two or three parts. There's no need to digest it all at once. When you find it difficult to focus on what's being suggested, that's a good time to take a break.

Lie on your back in a comfortably supported position. Have a small lift under your neck and head to assure that your airway is free. A bolster under your knees can ease tension in your lower back in this position. Close your eyes if that's comfortable for you.

Om

If you've ever attended a yoga class, you've probably encountered the custom of chanting the sound "om." Such chanting generally imparts a sense of peace and communal connection.

This syllable is mentioned in ancient mystical texts as early as the sixth century BCE and has been associated with various Hindu, Buddhist, and Sikh traditions. The sound may refer to the self or soul within, to cosmic truth, or to divine oneness.

The next time you have the opportunity of chanting—and right now might be as good a time as any—notice the reverberation of the sound throughout your fascial body. Your interoception lets you feel it all the way down to your soles. The phenomenon is particularly noticeable when you get to the humming at the end of the syllable. You may even begin to notice this fascial resonance when you are simply speaking. Besides putting you in touch with your fascial wholeness, humming, chanting, and singing help slow your breathing and raise vagal tone.

PRACTICE

Restful Breathing Meditation

🔊 **Practice 29 - Restful Breathing Meditation**

Surrender your weight into the surface on which you are lying. Feel the weight of your head, your chest, your pelvis, thighs, calves, and heels. Surrender your upper arms, elbows, forearms, and palms. Let your internal organs rest within your torso. Let your eyes settle back into their sockets.

Each time you exhale, let your body descend ever more deeply into the ground. Your diaphragm and your body as a whole relax together as you exhale.

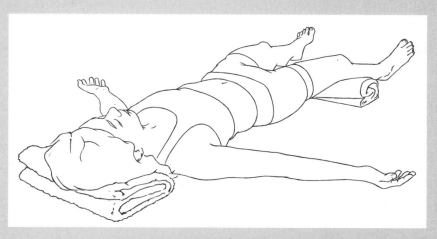

Beginning position for this exercise.

Become aware of a short pause at the end of your exhalation. This is a natural hiatus before you take your next breath. It is an emptying, a vacation right in the middle of your life. It's a moment in which you surrender your breath.

This is also a moment of rest for your hardworking diaphragm. It allows time for the respiratory center in your brain to register your need for more oxygen. The pause in your breath is fundamental to your being.

Each pause has its own integrity, its own right length of time. By letting the pause occur, you can welcome each breath as it emerges from the stillness. You don't have to reach for your breath. You simply open and allow the air to enter.

Now you can begin to notice the way the movement of your breathing affects the rest of your body. Imagine your body-wide mesh of fascial tissues, with quivering membranes and jelly-like pouches. Imagine your fascia as a soft and silky sponge. This tissue swells and settles with each cycle of your breath.

Picture your skeleton, your bones gliding within the fascial webbing. Each bone is independent—no bone touches another. As you breathe in and out, your bones seem to drift apart, and then together. You can sense that in your ankles. Your feet seem to slide away from your lower legs, opening the space within your ankle joints.

Notice how your pelvic bones subtly widen and narrow as your breath goes in and out.

Imagine the venetian blinds of your rib cage. The ribs tip upward and downward as you breathe in and breathe out. This natural breathing movement makes your rib cage wider side-to-side. And deeper front-to-back. Breathing this way helps you remember that you are a three-dimensional being.

As you inhale and your rib cage widens, the very tops of your upper arms roll slightly outward in their sockets. As you exhale, your upper arms roll inward. This motion is so subtle that you may think you are imagining it.

Your collarbones rise and spread apart while you inhale. And then they yield and descend.

You can sense your face widening with the inhalation, as if your cheekbones are moving apart, making more space for your nose and more space for your tongue. When you exhale, the back of your head yields more deeply into the ground. Your cheeks soften, and your lower jawbone descends.

Your fascial body ebbs and flows, emptying and filling like a sponge. Every cell in your body is breathing.

To conclude the practice, take time to become aware of your surroundings. Notice sounds outside the room. Then let your eyes open. Mindfully follow any impulse to move and stretch your body as you return to the "real world."

Take time to rise to a standing position. See whether you can feel some of the breathing movements that you noticed lying down. Sense your fascia responding to those movements. Sense your bones floating within your fascial body. How is it for you to be present with these sensations?

Review of Rolling Practice

At this point, it would be beneficial to return to the *Rolling* practice from chapter 2, to integrate your deepened awareness of your breath into that meditation. Then review *Rolling to Sidesaddle* from chapter 4 to practice breathing in the midst of activity.

Holding one's breath can be a way of feeling stable in unfamiliar circumstances, or when doing something new. *Rolling to Sidesaddle* was probably new for you the first time around, and you might have held your breath in an effort to get it right. Now, however, you're more familiar with the exercise. Match your breathing to the rhythm of the movement in a way that feels comfortable. Experiment with it. The support of the ground and the rise of bregma into the space give you balance and stability.

As always, take a walk. Breathing awareness is one of the surest ways to be in contact with your wholeness of being. The sentient, interoceptive capacity of your fascia grounds this in physical reality. As you walk around—ideally outdoors in a natural environment—you may have a clearer impression of yourself as a presence among other presences—what I was hinting at in chapter 2. Your own breath blesses you with that.

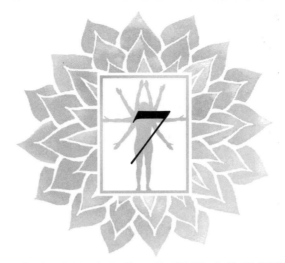

EMBODYING STRUCTURE

[In organisms] what are called structures are actually slow processes of long duration, while functions are quick processes of short duration. Thus, if we say that a function, such as the contraction of a muscle, is performed by a structure, it means that a quick and short process wave is superimposed on a long-lasting and slowly running wave.

LUDWIG VON BERTALANFFY, AUSTRIAN BIOLOGIST
AND NOBEL LAUREATE, *PROBLEMS OF LIFE,* 1952

Ida P. Rolf, Ph.D.

Ida P. Rolf, Ph.D., mentioned in chapter 1 as the founder of the manual therapy she called Structural Integration, was responsible for two ideas about the body that were revolutionary for the mid-twentieth century. First, she taught that human bodies are as affected by the force of gravity as are nonliving architectural structures. People didn't think about bodies as structures in those days. Rolf's architecture metaphor was a simple way to demonstrate gravity's influence. Your body is a house: pain and poor posture are like door hinges that squeak because the foundation has settled unevenly.

REFLECTION
Perfectly Balanced—Perfectly Crooked

I have a good eye for structural imbalances. I can identify the off-kilter details that explain idiosyncrasies in how people move. Watching pedestrians in crosswalks, I filter my vision because otherwise their midlines look unbearably fragmented to me, their bodies painfully crooked.

I can also tell you a lot about my own crookedness.

Although it wouldn't be obvious to most observers, I bear more weight on my left foot than my right. The left side of my pelvis torques back, and my left sacroiliac joint is stiff. Fascia on the left side of my lumbar spine is thicker than on the right. My ribs are closer together on the left, and my left shoulder blade tucks into my rib cage. From its base at the top of my shoulders, my neck angles to the right, counterbalancing the leftward lean of everything below. The compression on the left side shunts my pelvis to the right, making my right hip unstable.

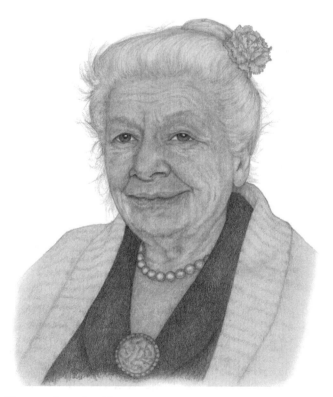

Ida P. Rolf, Founder of Rolfing Structural Integration. Drawing based on a photograph by Ron Thompson and used with his permission.

In assessing where all those parts are relative to each other, I've "read" my body using my proprioception. The reading depends on conceiving of my body as parts. It's based on a compression model of structure. Proprioception divorced from deeper interoceptive sensing seduces me into manipulating my body image. When I am persuaded by this appeal to my perfectionism, I become deaf to deeper voices within my body, within myself.

———

Rolf's second revolutionary idea was that human structures could change for the better. Until then, it had been assumed that the set of your shoulders and the flatness of your feet were genetic givens. You had your father's feet and your grandmother's shoulders, and that was that.

Rolf understood fascia to be a continuous tissue medium that contained and buttressed structure.

She saw that it hardened in response to the stress of imbalance and compression. Since imbalanced posture deformed the fascia, it stood to reason that fascia, and hence posture, could be reshaped. Her approach was to apply energy to the fascia by means of touch. She observed that touch often affected the body at some distance, from the place being touched, and deduced that forces were conducted through the fascia. Since that time, it has been proposed that fascia may indeed conduct bioelectricity, although the amount of electricity generated by touch is probably minimal. So we still do not know how the global effects of Structural Integration bodywork are achieved, although the recently discovered sensory capacity of fascia may unlock this mystery.

The logo Ida Rolf chose for her work shows a little boy with poor posture juxtaposed with an imbalanced stack of blocks. Next to this figure is a child with balanced posture shown against a plumb line. The logo reveals Rolf's adherence to the accepted Newtonian view of body mechanics. This view likens the body to a building constructed of vertical posts and horizontal beams. The building's components are held together by the compressive force of gravity. In the logo, the plumb line represents gravity. This is a mechanical model of the body. In part 1 of this book, you applied this model to yourself during the preparatory body reading.

A mechanical body model achieves motion by means of levers and hinges, and bones and joints neatly fit those categories. Muscles are like motors attached to the bony levers.

When I studied with her, Rolf taught us to assess a body's structure against a visualized grid of vertical and horizontal lines. Joints were explained as hinges whose actions were to be adjusted along vertical and horizontal axes. We learned to manipulate the fascia until we could imagine perpendicular lines in the tissue. For example, if a client carried one shoulder higher than the other, he likely displayed oblique lines through the upper chest. We used our hands to "horizontalize" the tissues of the rib cage, shoulder, and spine, thereby improving the functioning of all those joints.

Rolf's system of bodywork assessment and technique was, and still is, effective, but classical geometry explains her method only to a limited extent. Bodies aren't made of vertical posts and horizontal crossbeams. But of course she knew that.

Tensegrity

In the 1960s Rolf became familiar with the concept of **tensegrity**, a term coined by Buckminster Fuller, American architect, systems theorist, and inventor of the geodesic dome. Fuller's term refers to the *tensional integrity* achieved through balance between tension and compression. In a tensegrity structure, rigid struts are

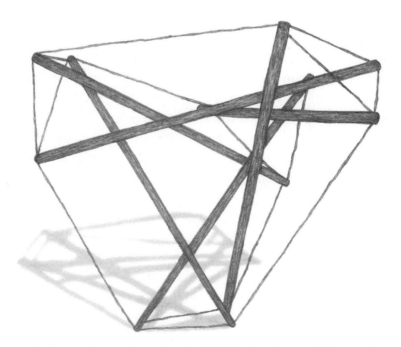

A structure similar to the one here inspired Fuller's coinage of the word tensegrity.
A large and extensive tensegrity structure, called "Needle Tower,"
by artist Kenneth Snelson, can be seen at the National Mall in Washington, DC.

suspended between tensioned cables or, in the case of the body, tensioned soft tissue. Tensegrity was a helpful metaphor for Rolf because it allowed the body to be conceived as spacious rather than solid. But the tensile characteristic of fascia wasn't consistent with the compressive model of structure. In a block model, fascia was seen as a kind of glue that hardened when the stack of blocks was out of alignment. Tensegrity was a better fit for Rolf's theory because it understood fascia as a changeable and responsive element in structural organization.

Developing her work in the period prior to significant fascia research, Rolf had it both ways: the body was a stack of blocks *and* a tensegrity structure. Thanks to her genius as a manual therapist, she was able to communicate her vision despite its theoretical inconsistencies and to inspire several generations of practitioners. The Ida Rolf Foundation is a major sponsor of the Fascial Research Congresses, and in this way her inquiry into the nature of human structure continues.

Biotensegrity

Thanks to the collective creativity of fascial research scientists, bodily organization is now being further reconceived as **biotensegrity** (a term coined by orthopedic surgeon Stephen Levin).

To understand the difference between tensegrity and biotensegrity, consider a camping tent. A dome tent is organized by tensegrity. Stiff rods are held in place by flexible fabric. The tension and compression parts of the structure are connected but are essentially distinct. If you remove the rods, the fabric, being inert, will sag, and your tent will collapse. Conversely, should the fabric somehow vanish, the rods would clatter to the ground. Further, a tensegrity structure, necessarily tethered to the ground, cannot move on its own.

Like all vertebrates, our bodies are designed for movement. Survival is determined by mobility. Our bodies cannot depend, like a tent does, on external support. We must be self-supporting, able to sustain our coherence whether or not our feet are planted on the ground.

In a biotensegrity structure, the tension and compression members are considered to be different manifestations of the same basic material. Bones are denser than the elastic fascial continuum that surrounds them but are made of essentially the same stuff. Rather than coordinating movement through a sequence of levered joint actions, bones transmit movement by means of shifting tensional polarities that involve the entire fascial network. Each joint's slightest adjustment affects the whole to some degree. And because the whole is elastic, the body's structural integrity remains constant throughout movement.

After a moment of shock and tears, a healthy child bounces back from a slip and fall. For an older person whose habits of movement have confined his fascial system to a hinged compression arrangement, a similar fall can result in serious injury and lasting distortion of structure. By providing a whole-body response to any local mechanical stress, along with return to the original shape, biotensegrity affords your body a degree of independence from the force of gravity.

In chapter 4, you were able to reach passionately for something in "the upper-right corner" without destroying your integrity. Your whole body shape-shifted in response to change in the angle of the struts and the pull on the fabric, and shape-shifted again when you brought your arm down. Your "body tent" did not collapse because your fascia is not inert; it is responsive, living tissue.

If you must rest a broken arm in a sling for a month, your fascia redistributes the tensions throughout your body so you can stay balanced and stable while you recover. Once the break has healed, your tensegrity must be reconfigured. The more mobile your lifestyle, the easier this is. Active children, for example, reorganize themselves quickly. But in the Digital Age, most adults' movements have little variety. Consequently, a month in a cast can leave a strong sensory imprint and generate compensatory fascial shadows across distant areas of the body. Therapy that addresses only the muscles of the injured limb doesn't impact the entire body. We recover but may never feel quite whole again.

Our movements result from the combined forces of muscular contraction and fascial transmission. In real life, muscles don't contract in isolation the way we're told they do in a gym. Instead, portions of muscles go on line in sequence, depending on the type of movement being performed. The movements of life rarely occur in a single plane. The biceps brachii muscles can certainly flex the lower arm toward the upper arm, which makes the elbow *seem* to be a lever. But in real-life arm activity, portions of the biceps partner with portions of many other muscles to produce movements that occur in many planes at once.

Consider the elbow movement of a tennis serve: muscles and fascial elements that weave around the elbow produce motions that can occur simultaneously in three planes. Such movements are spiralic rather than hinged. Further, they occur congruently with the spiraling action of the whole body in the serve. Integrating the varying pulls of all the involved muscles, fascia's elasticity broadly distributes power. Fascia also distributes sensory feedback, so the athlete may intuit the success of the serve long before the ball lands.

When we observe elegant, resilient movement, our mirror neurons recognize it. Our bodies respond when we watch a couple dancing a tango or a basketball player's elegant dunk. We feel pleasure, enthusiasm, even kinship. As we watch these biotensegrities in motion, we recognize beauty. Humanity.

A lever-and-hinges style of movement evokes quite different emotions. The street dance known as "animation" both amuses and unnerves us because it is incongruent to see a human moving in such a nonhuman manner. The mechanical, nontensegral motion of soldiers marching in unison inspires fear or patriotism depending on how people feel about armies. The awkwardly hinged movement of a person with a disability (like Ian Waterman, mentioned in chapter 1) may cause us to recoil or to reach out with compassion.

The concept of biotensegrity as an organizing principle of human structure mirrors the organization of our microanatomy. Fascia researcher Donald Ingber, MD, shows that tensegrity architecture organizes not only our bodily shape, but everything within our bodies, from tissues and organs to molecules and cells.[1] Each time you move, the mechanical forces being transmitted through your body are converted into chemical changes within your cells. This process—called **mechanotransduction**—even affects the expression of your genes. Ingber's work suggests how deeply our bodies are affected by how (or whether) we move them.

Jean-Claude Guimberteau, whose beautiful images of living fascia you saw in chapter 1, regards tensegrity as a good theoretical model to explain how the seemingly chaotic fascial universe within our bodies is ordered. But although fascia research has brought us closer to understanding the human body, much remains for us to learn about our miraculous organism.

I'm dealing with problems in the body where there is never just one cause.
I'd like you to have more reality on the circular processes that do not act
in the body but are the body. The body process is not linear: it is circular;
always it is circular. One thing goes awry and its effects go on and on and
on and on. A body is a web connecting everything with everything else.[2]

IDA P. ROLF, PH.D.

Tensegral Expansion

In chapters 3 and 4, you began experiencing the way your awareness of the space around your body affects your posture. Freedom to move through any trajectory, from any point on or within your body, results in an open and expanded bodily shape. Thus, *awareness of the space around your body helps maintain the space within your body.* I think of this as tensegrity of perception. It is as if your body is suspended and supported within an invisible network of potential vectors.

Expansive body use decompresses your joints and adjusts fascial tensions to engage all elements in your personal biotensegrity. Your body feels bigger, more open, and more vibrant. You take up more space on the outside and have more room on the inside.

When your entire body shares the shifting loads, everything participates in support of the whole, and nothing collapses or buckles. Your struts and elastic tissues are all equally involved in your coordination, which gives your movement an elegant flow. Your body's **tensegral expansion** primes your fascia's energy storage capacity so you can be ready to spring into action.

Tensegral body attitude, by expanding the space within the torso, grants more living room to your organs, beneficially affecting all visceral functions, including circulation, respiration, and digestion. And, because expansive visceral space contributes to high vagal tone, it can positively affect both health and social connectedness. In other words, an open body attitude contributes to an open perspective on life.

When you are oriented spatially in three dimensions, that orientation helps support your body as a mobile biotensegrity. As a biotensegrity creature, you change shape organically, responding to what you feel within yourself and sense in the space around you. A sedentary lifestyle diminishes your perception of your surroundings. With reduced experience of inner and outer spatial expansion, your body assumes the compression model of structure. The downside of fascia is that immobility makes it fibrous and dense. Not only does immobility predispose your body to poor posture, stiff, awkward movement, and injury, it also reduces your capacity for expression. *You live yourself into the shapes that you most often assume.*

Lifestyle that includes the right kinds of movement keeps fascia healthy, resilient, and adaptable. Whole-body movement through many vectors in space, movement that is nonhabitual and in which you participate with active awareness—not on autopilot—engages your tensegrity. When you can be dually oriented to ground and space, your **perceptual tensegrity** facilitates your expression of tensegral movement.

Spatial Medicine

Thomas Myers, anatomist and author of *Anatomy Trains,* has coined the term "spatial medicine" to designate "healing through rearranging the body in space."[3] Attending to the conformation of the space within the body is a very different approach from the conventional medical model that emphasizes healing through chemical means. Practitioners of spatial medicine include not only specialists in Rolf's Structural Integration but also massage therapists, osteopaths, chiropractors, yoga and Pilates teachers, personal trainers, athletics coaches, dance and martial arts instructors, and even orthopedic surgeons—in short, anyone concerned with optimizing human form and movement. Many of these professionals do not yet realize their shared synergistic and holistic view of the body. Research into fascia, neural plasticity, biotensegrity, and human movement offers cross-pollination among the branches of spatial medicine.

Power Posing

Reading another person's facial expression or body language to predict their behavior is something we all do to some degree. Panhandlers assess our potential for compassion or guilt, and we ourselves wait until a friend seems relaxed and receptive before asking them for a favor.

Harvard social scientist Amy Cuddy suggests that the reverse is also true: our own body language can change our feelings about ourselves, our behavior, and even our physiology. Her studies followed volunteers who assumed expanded body positions for two minutes and were then found to be more open to risk-taking than were volunteers who sat curled up with their arms folded across their torsos. Further, people who spent two minutes in expansive postures prior to mock job interviews were judged to be enthusiastic, authentic, comfortable, confident, and generally more "present" than volunteers who had assumed closed, nonpowerful postures before the interview. Cuddy's study also showed that what she terms "power posing" changes hormone levels, lowering the stress hormone, cortisol, and raising the dominance hormone, testosterone. Typical power poses include raising the arms up in a V, like an athlete's gesture of victory, or standing with arms akimbo—hands on the hips.

Although Cuddy's findings on hormone fluctuations have yet to be definitively proven, her work suggests that positive biochemical effects could also be expected from regular awareness and practice of tensegral expansion. Cuddy's 2012 TED talk, "Your Body Language May Shape Who You Are," had received, as of this writing, over 43 million views. Such popularity reflects, I believe, not only hunger for success but also a drive to feel more comfortable and whole in our bodies.

Re-assess Your Stance

The following exploration is an opportunity to compare your impression of your standing posture with the body reading you did at the beginning of *Body Mandala*. If you do this exploration with closed eyes, your sensory impressions will be more intense. To feel safe, stand near a wall in case your balance becomes unsteady. Remember that feeling sensations and imagining sensations both occur in your brain's sensory cortex. If you think you're just imagining things, go right ahead.

PRACTICE

Re-assess Your Stance

◀)) Practice 30 - Re-assess Your Stance

Stand comfortably with your weight evenly distributed between your feet. You may notice that your upright stance wavers a bit. Let yourself appreciate that subtle motion. This is a normal **postural sway** through which your nerves, muscles, and fascia negotiate your decision to stand in one place.

Close your eyes to gather a more distinct impression of the natural sway that occurs at your ankle joints. Remind yourself of the presence of your midline. Let it extend downward through your perineal point to the ground and upward through your crown point to the sky. Expanding your midline will help you sense the postural sway throughout your body.

Feel—or imagine feeling—the ends of your lower leg bones softly moored in the fascial matrix that separates them from your feet. Then trace the swaying sensation upward through your lower legs, into your knees. Soften your knees, so your thighbones can be poised above your shins without compressing your knee joints.

Then bring your awareness farther up until you feel your pelvis suspended over the ball bearings of your hip joints. Feel the subtle sway of your hips and pelvis, the sway of your spine.

Now, become aware of the movement of breathing throughout your fascial body—imagine the tiny opalescent fibers changing shape. You can feel the whole-body expansion that occurs when you inhale. The ground welcomes your feet, while the air caresses your skin.

Continue appreciating your sensations and open your eyes.

Imagine yourself waiting in line in an everyday situation. Imagine yourself taking a moment to tune into these body phenomena, right in the middle of your busy day.

During this process—it will be slightly different each time you do it—you may notice contrasts between the way you experience your body on the left side and on the right, in front and in back, upper body and lower.

Notice where you feel the aliveness of your tissues most intensely, where it's easiest to sense the movement of your breath, where your body feels dense or spacious, dull or vibrant. Observe such contrasts without concern and without attempting to improve your posture by changing what you feel. Simply feel. Let any meaning that might be associated with your sensations be a product of spontaneous discovery rather than a mental hunting expedition.

Asymmetrical Stance

Early in part 1, I invited you to notice which leg you lift first when you put on your pants. This mundane habitual movement reflects a subtle body-wide imbalance of fascial tension, probably developed over decades. It tweaks your tensegrity to such a degree that even when you think you have your weight evenly balanced on both legs, you probably don't. In the moment right before you move, you will stabilize yourself by a slight loading of what I call your "preferred leg."

Contrapposto or "counterpose" is an Italian term used in sculpture to describe a human figure standing with most of his or her weight on one leg and with the upper body twisting contralaterally to the pelvis and legs. Michelangelo's famous *David* is a Renaissance interpretation of a common ancient Greek theme of the heroic male. Contrapposto is considered by art authorities to be a visually harmonious portrayal of a calm mental state. It also represents beauty.

However, if we consider this biblical hero from a structural point of view, we can assume that he raises his left leg first when he pulls on his boots. The entire right side of his body is compressed, and this compression would have been reflected in his gait. Once his warrior days were over, he may have developed a bit of arthritis in his right knee. This is silly, of course, but the serious point is that media (statues were the media of the ancients) distorts our perception of what is beautiful, healthy, strong, and serene. You'll see contrapposto throughout the pages of *Vanity Fair* or *People* magazines. If you look carefully, you'll also see that most people's gait is slightly asymmetrical.

If you haven't identified your "preferred leg," do that now. Which of your feet lifts first to pass through the leg of your jeans? The other leg is your preferred one—you rely on it for stability and balance.

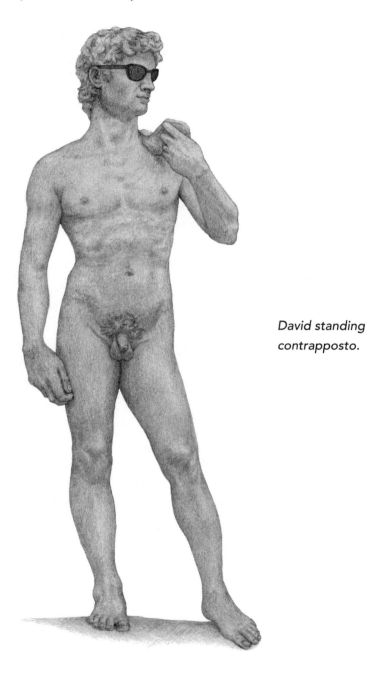

David standing contrapposto.

Try this additional test: stand relaxed and still, and then step forward as if someone has called your name. Most likely you will begin by shifting your weight to the preferred side and swinging the other leg forward first. Reversing the forward step will feel oddly unfamiliar.

How you step into your jeans can become a practical cue to tune up your tensegrity. To do so, you have to be present in your body. Initially it won't be easy to yield the weight of your body into your less-stable side. You'll need to recall your midline polarity and tap into your awareness of peripersonal space. The attempt to change this mundane habit every morning can be a daily reminder of your postural pattern as a whole. The more you remember it, the easier it becomes to decompress your body throughout the day.

Other Stabilizing Habits

Hopefully, the Body Mandala explorations have begun to change the way you conceive of your posture by understanding it as a vast network of intelligent and communicating tissues. You have begun to sense yourself as being organized through multidirectional tensions within your body, and by potential vectors in the space around your body. You are a biotensegrity being, but also a perceptual tensegrity being, structured by the way you relate to the ground and to your surroundings. And, at times, when under stress, you may also find yourself to be compressed like a stack of blocks.

Inspirational as it may be to reconceive ourselves as biotensegrities, the habit of compression dies hard. Imbalanced posture is a loss of tensegrity in part or all of the structure. Under stress, we seem to revert to the mechanical version of our bodies. Weak areas, no longer supported by the whole, begin to buckle. Creatures of expediency, we vacillate between our options.

Many tension patterns are simple habits, like putting on your pants the same way for years. Others are complex strategies for feeling safe in circumstances that echo historical situations in which we have felt unsafe. They're successful strategies—they wouldn't have become habits if they hadn't worked. But usually they are anachronisms, no longer pertinent to our present time selves.

PRACTICE

A Stabilization Scenario

🔊 **Practice 31 - A Stabilization Scenario**

Begin by standing comfortably and breathing for several moments.

Then call to mind something you've been concerned about—a miscommunication with someone, a deadline, a health issue. You may immediately notice how that concern affects your tissues—how it affects your shape, affects the ease of your respiration.

Imagine you are waiting for important news, and the telephone rings.

What do you sense in your body in the nanoseconds just before you step out to reach for the phone?

My own postural imbalances alert me to the probability that I've mentally strayed from the present moment. I know that I lean to the left when I'm tired or sad and compress my chest when I try hard to get something done. As you become better acquainted with your own stabilizing patterns, you'll begin to receive your own "somatic alerts."

The practice on this page invites you to imagine a scenario that can help you identify another of your stabilizing habits. For the scene, you will need a phone, but put it across the room, not in your pocket. Before you begin, walk around in an easy way to establish a neutral body attitude.

Every step you take requires a moment of stabilization. Ideally, your sense of being supported by the ground and oriented in space primes your body with tensegral expansion, letting you move forward with balance and ease. But when you're stressed, even a little, you likely rely on habits of stabilizing yourself that are compressive rather than expansive.

Consider what you felt in your body right before you reached out to grasp the phone. Was it a familiar sensation? It could have manifested as a barely perceptible narrowing of your chest, ducking of your head, or raising of your shoulders. Less obvious gestures might be a subtle gripping of your toes, or a barely noticeable clenching of your jaw or palms.

Whatever your pattern might be, it is an attempt to buttress yourself against possible bad news.

Somewhere in your body, your tissues hardened. In that moment your trust in the ground eroded and your awareness of your surroundings dimmed. You held yourself together without the aid of your perceptions. You became a stack of blocks.

Most of us have numerous stabilizing strategies. You'll need to be a bit like Sherlock Holmes to ferret them out. It helps that you're ramping up your interoception through the explorations in this book. As you become more sentient and feel more centered and more whole, awkward body responses will be easier to discern.

In terms of your Body Mandala, your stabilizing patterns are tiny moments of self-expression, products of sensation and movement. Mapped in your brain and fixed in your fascia, they remain unconscious. Over time, such anticipatory movements solidify into distortions of structure, further restricting your freedom of expression. Your Body Mandala practice interrupts this vicious circle.

Poor stabilization habits often prevail in moments of impatience or frustration when you feel that time is slipping by too fast. Breath holding, after either inhalation or exhalation, is a common stabilizing habit. It is as if, by not breathing, you think you are controlling time. Even happiness can create patterns of tension. In anticipation of a happy outcome, it's common for your sense of relationship to the ground to evaporate. You may be surprised at the extent to which you recruit your stabilization strategies for the most mundane circumstances.

Your posture is quite the opposite of a static, finished position. It is a dynamic activity, characterized by changes in your perceptions, in your outlook and expression, in the tone of your fascia, in the state of your nervous system, in the responsiveness of your cells. You are an organism, not a set of components or a stack of bricks.

Embryonic Midline

Ida Rolf's writings emphasized that the human body's central axis is a consequence of gravitation. Among her students, however, she acknowledged that other energies were at play. "Rolfers," she said, ". . . so organize the body that the gravity field can reinforce the body's energy field."[4]

The vertical line has been a symbol of human aspiration for millennia. It's portrayed as the Tree of Life, as Jacob's ladder, as the Christian cross, as the movement of powerful kundalini energy in the Indian spiritual tradition. A possible explanation for the potency of the central line as a symbol is found in the field of embryology.

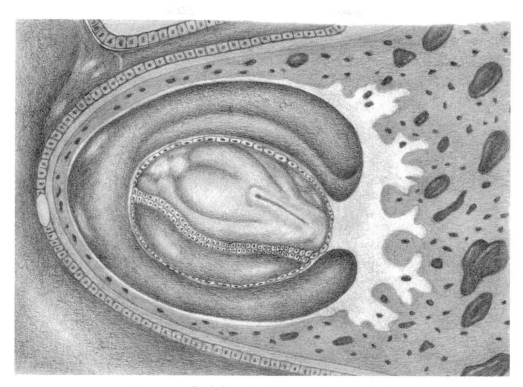

*A seam called the primitive streak appears in
embryonic tissue fifteen days after conception*

A longitudinal seam, called the **primitive streak**, appears in embryonic tissue a mere fifteen days after conception. This transient streak grows upward through a disc-like formation of fascial tissue, establishing a top and bottom, left and right. Thus, we are spatially oriented long before we are fully formed. The streak is the precursor of the spinal cord and spine. For the next five weeks, the developing tissue expands, folds, twists in upon itself, opens out again, and refolds like origami, forming new layers, chambers, and protrusions. At the end of eight weeks, the folding tissue has become an embryo. Such creation is no stacking of parts, no assembling of levers. It is a dance of tensegral expansion.[5]

Some osteopathic physicians believe that the embryonic midline kindles our aliveness throughout our days, influencing the health of body, mind, and spirit. Awareness of the polarity between bregma and your perineal point is a physical metaphor for this generative midline.

REFLECTION
Toweling Off

On busy days, a morning shower can be my biggest luxury. The soothing, streaming water is hypnotic—it's precious time away from it all. But the moment I step on the bathmat, real life crashes in, urging me to get dry and get on with it. I'm already *there* in my head, as distinct from being *here* in my body.

One day I conceive a rationale—if one were needed—for continuing to luxuriate.

Toweling off is opportunity to activate my skin's tactile sensors, to remind my skin to feel its interface with the air. My towel awakens interoceptive sensors in the fascia beneath my skin. Interoception is a very big deal, a capacity most of us need to revive. I've written a whole book, largely about that.

So I take three extra minutes to *enjoy* toweling off, to let my skin take in the sensations of the fabric, and to appreciate the rhythm and pressure of my contact with myself. I pause. My brain needs a moment to convert my utilitarian drying-off motions into an interoceptive experience of opening to the contact with my own touch.

I think about Sensei, leisurely grooming himself, intent on each tongue-stroke of fur, not needing to be reminded that his body and mind are one. But I must work to keep my attention trained on the interface between my skin and the towel. I try new angles, different strokes, aware that I'm refreshing my sense of bodily self.

Once dry, I pause for a moment more, sensing the air against my skin boundary, noticing how my skin abuts the space in all directions. I imagine tiny vectors extending out into space from every pore. At the same time, I feel my body resting down, supported by the floor. I coin a phrase to describe the experience: **perceptual tensegrity.**

I feel bigger, fuller, and, curiously, less tilted to the left. It's a fine way to start the day.

SENTIENT FOUNDATIONS

They paved paradise
And put up a parking lot

JONI MITCHELL

What Is a Foot?

It's a common assumption that the foot is poorly designed—that it's too rigid and too delicate to form the human body's foundation. This seems to be borne out by the statistic that 75 percent of people in the United States have foot pain at some time in their lives.[1] But it's the mechanical view of body structure that relegates feet to the bottom of the block pile. The conception of the body as a biotensegrity requires that we adjust our assumptions about our feet. This will also change our understanding of foot problems.

When you've been standing on them all day long, it can be all too evident that your feet are structural support elements. But they are not platforms propping up a stack of blocks. Inherent in, and crucial to, your tensional integrity, they communicate with your entire structure as you walk and move. Underactive, toneless feet put a drag on the whole tensegrity structure; rigid feet keep it strung too tightly.

Poorly supportive feet aren't necessarily sore feet, however. Because your fascial network is adaptive, poor foot support can be expressed in other areas of the body. Tight shoulders, for example, can be a way of lifting the body up from feet that don't provide a good foundation. Imbalance and pain in the neck can result from an imbalanced or nonresilient foot. Conversely, mobility and resilience in the feet contribute to body-wide fascial balance, and to the ease and freedom of everything above them.

In addition to their supportive role, feet are complex *sense organs*. There are 200,000 nerve endings in the soles of your feet. That means that your body is equipped to receive a great deal of information through your relationship to the ground. In your brain, the sensory representation of your feet is almost as great as that of your hands, lips, and genitals. Feet can gauge terrain for secure purchase, respond to thorns and pebbles with tiny adjustments to balance, and gather other sensory information that we wearers of shoes can hardly imagine. Eons ago, a bare foot meeting the earth might read the morning news through touch, literally sensing the activities of other creatures in the neighborhood.

There are twenty-six bones in each foot, each tiny bone suspended in gel-like fascia. Interstices between the bones make up thirty-three joints—in each foot. More than a hundred muscles, tendons, and ligaments give these joints potential to move. The sole of the foot is cushioned with a fat-infused fascial layer, the so-called "fat pad," that helps dampen both vertical impact and lateral pressures on the sole of the foot. The complexity of the foot's design suggests that it should be able to conform to the contours and textures of varied terrains.

With each step your foot's adaptation to the ground is transmitted upward through the fascia of your leg into your pelvis and lower back. This means there's a direct relationship between movements your feet make and the mobility of your body as a whole. Each foot is a complex tensegrity structure in and of itself, as well as being integral to the tensegrity of the body above. If the foot is too lax or too stiff, then tensegrity is cut off at the ankles.

Because biologic structure is dynamic—not a stacking of objects, but a constantly morphing interplay of tensional relationships—it's only logical that structural foundations must also be dynamic.

Ancestral Feet

For nearly six million years, human feet walked through grassy meadows, across pine needle forest floors, and over volcanic rock. But, for the last several millennia, our feet have been shod, encased in what my colleague Dr. Phillip Beach calls "sensory deprivation chambers."[2] Further, thanks to the industrial revolution and the automobile, feet have been further desensitized by the convenience of walking on hard, flat, unvarying surfaces. Rarely do modern feet have opportunity to express their innate potential for mobility and sensory intelligence.

Sensitivity Training for Your Feet

The adaptability of your structure as a whole is married to the adaptability of your feet. Given the intercommunicative nature of your fascial system, heightening awareness in your feet will beneficially affect the tone and function of your entire body. Indeed, finding your footing—*embodying* your footing—is essential to maintaining healthy posture and movement.

Practices in this chapter help you sense the profound relationship between your feet and the rest of your body. You begin by using the sensitivity of your hands to remind your feet how much they, too, can feel.

PRACTICE

Interoceptive Hands Meditation

🔊 **Practice 32 - Interoceptive Hands Meditation**

Standing comfortably, bring your palms together at waist level, thumbs and fingers pointing away from your body. Without pressing hard, make complete

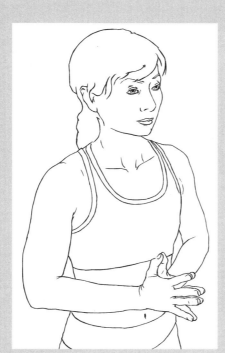

Position of hands for Interoceptive Hands Meditation.

contact between the entire skin surface of your fingers and palms. Your eyes may be closed or open with a soft focus.

As you become aware of the ebb and flow of your breathing throughout your body, begin to imagine your bones gliding in their bed of fascia. They float inside your body, and yet they have weight. Sense the weight in your pelvic bones, your shins, and the weight of the knobs on both sides of each ankle. These are your **malleoli**—feel how heavy they are. Feel the broad footprints your feet are making on the floor.

Feel your rib cage as it widens and settles with your breathing. Feel the weight of your shoulder blades and let them slide down along your back. Become aware of the aliveness of your hands.

Now, appreciate the obvious—that your right hand is touching the left, and that your left hand is receiving sensation from the right. You feel this as a flow of sensation rather than as muscular activity. Consider whether the direction of that sensory flow from right to left feels familiar.

Now reverse the flow. Become aware that your left hand can give sensation to the right, and that your right hand can be receptive. There's no muscular effort in your arms or shoulders because the tactile exchange takes place in your brain. But you may feel an expanding sensation in your left arm. Your right hand is open and relaxed as it receives sensation. Observe whether the sensory flow from left to right feels familiar.

Focus on the communication of aliveness between your hands, as they take turns giving and receiving sensation. Pause briefly each time you reverse the flow. As your hands trade roles, you may sense subtle changes elsewhere in your fascial body.

When you are ready, relax your hands at your sides, letting them remain present in the background of your awareness.

While offered as preparation for the foot practice that follows, you may want to take some time to integrate the *Interoceptive Hands Meditation*. It's fine to postpone the foot meditation for another session. Take a walk. Appreciate the effect that sensory awakening of your hands has had on your posture, your coordination, and your point of view.

PRACTICE

Interoceptive Feet Meditation

◀)) Practice 33 - Interoceptive Feet Meditation

Stand comfortably in bare feet. Remember your midline. Let your eyes have a soft focus.

With hands together, briefly refresh the sensory communication between your hands.

Now, transfer the experience of your hands to the contact between your feet and the ground. Become aware of the way each foot touches the ground.

Let your feet be generous—all toes present, arches present, heels present. As you inhale, your body opens, and your soles seem to spread into the ground.

As you exhale, each foot receives the weight of your body and senses the certainty of the ground. Savor these impressions. Continue for several breathing cycles—inhaling and touching the ground, then exhaling and letting the ground receive you through your feet.

From there, begin a gentle sideways sway. Let your midline drift an inch or two to the right. Your body's weight shifts onto the outside edge of your right foot and the inside edge of your left foot. Softly reverse the motion, now settling your weight into the outer edge of your left foot, and inner edge of your right foot. Continue swaying. Feel the effects of this small movement in your legs, hips, pelvis, and spine. Go slowly. You may notice the fascial interplay as far upward as your neck. Then bring yourself to center.

When you walk around after this practice, you may notice that the ground seems to rise up to meet your feet. This can be the beginning of a new relationship between the reality of the ground and the capacity of your feet to receive that reality.

> ### Anatomy Terms
>
> It's not necessary to remember all the anatomical terms I'm introducing in the discussion that follows. My aim in this section is to help you envision and experience the subtle motions of your feet.
>
> Anatomical descriptors are the easiest way for me to summarize the movements of the foot. Ordinary language would make the descriptions much more cumbersome.

Restoring sensory awareness to your feet can be a challenging process. Modern feet are sensation-deprived because they walk entirely on flat surfaces and because of the sensation-dulling effect of shoes. When humans stopped walking on dirt, we stopped using our feet as sense organs. This seems to have changed the collective body image of our species—feet became less integral to the body as a whole.

The distinction between the perception that your feet are *on the floor* and the perception that your feet are *receiving the floor* may be elusive at first. If so, keep coming back to this meditation. If receiving support from the ground is to become a felt experience rather than a concept, your brain has some changes to make. You may even be aware of a mild struggle in your brain, or moments of awkwardness when you move. Such moments indicate that your nervous system is trying to incorporate new sensations and movements. What your feet are learning challenges your brain's plasticity. Awkwardness can be a sign that your brain maps are being revised.

The new map takes time to develop. But you can practice at odd moments throughout the day—when standing in a line, for example. And be sure to incorporate your newly receptive feet into your yoga practice or gym workout.

Your Feet Are Propellers

If your skeleton as a whole is suspended in a foam of fascia, then that is also true of the fifty-two bones of your feet. They can't be excluded from the overall biotensegrity design. Like the rest of your body, your feet have the capacity for tensegral expansion.

To understand the internal workings of the foot, it's helpful to divide the foot into thirds: the back third includes the heel and anklebone; the middle third includes five small bones of the mid-foot, called *tarsals*. The front third, your forefoot, includes the five *metatarsal* bones and the toes. These "thirds" roughly correlate to the three phases of walking: heel contact, stance, and push-off. It's also helpful to imagine that each foot has a midline that runs from the center of your heel to the cleavage between your second and third toes.

You're probably familiar with the arch on the big toe side of each foot. Actually, each foot has three arches. The familiar one is the inner or *medial arch*. You also have a shallow arch along the outside edge of your foot, the *lateral arch,* and a *transverse arch* that runs across the middle third of your foot. Ideally, taking a step involves rotation around the foot's midline from the lateral arch across the transverse arch to the medial arch and back again. The inward turning motion is called **pronation**, and the outward turning motion is **supination**. By coordinating these motions, a well-functioning foot meets the ground with a subtle spiraling action, something like a propeller.

Between the back third and middle third of your foot is a crosswise joint, the *midtarsal joint.* It lies directly below where your shoelaces tie. The surfaces that compose this joint are rounded enough to allow pronation and supination around the midline. When you practiced the swaying motion of *Interoceptive Feet,* you were alternately pronating and supinating through your midtarsal joints. These micromovements should also occur in normal walking.

When you put your right heel down to take a step, there is a brief moment in which your weight rests onto your lateral arch. As your weight travels forward into the middle third of your foot—this is called the "stance phase" of your step—you pronate very slightly through the midtarsal joint as your weight shifts into your medial arch. The movement is an arc, a fragment of a spiral.

Let's say you've just now stepped onto your right heel and moved forward into the stance phase. During the nanosecond you're poised over the middle third of your right foot, your left leg initiates a swing forward to take the next step. As your left foot swings, your right foot pushes off through its front third. This involves a lightning-fast maneuver of the front third of your foot that tones the transverse arch and turns it into a miniature spring. This forefoot activity is the basis of a resilient push-off into the next step.

Modern humans don't require a dynamic push-off to traverse the confined spaces of contemporary life. Consequently we tend to underuse the front and middle thirds of our feet. This habit reduces tensegral expansion throughout the legs, pelvis, and spine.

High Arches and Flat Feet

If your feet have high, rigid arches, you will find it easy to rest into the lateral arches of your feet, but difficult to pronate—to feel your weight yielding into the medial arch. If your foot is quite pronated, it will be difficult for you to supinate without lifting your big toes from the ground. You'll find much more detail about foot patterns in *Know Your Feet,* my online workshop.* In it, you'll see and feel the details of foot design and mechanics, understand the interplay between the three arches, make a precise assessment of your own feet, and learn self-care exercises tailored to flat feet and high, rigid arches.

Activate Your Forefeet

Before hominids developed upright walking, a foot could wrap itself around a rock or a tree branch and use that purchase to push off from. Prehensile feet actively interacted with the environment. Feet reached out to clasp each next point of security, alternately opening and grasping as they moved through canopy or across terrain. Modern feet retain that ability to clasp, but our use of it is more nuanced. Clasping survives as a toning of the forefoot that precedes push-off. It provides the spring in our steps.

Contemporary walking takes place on hard, flat, unvarying surfaces and in confined environments that do not inspire use of our bodies' fascial elasticity and tensegral expansion. Resilient push-off becomes redundant. But, when the forefoot is never activated, over time the transverse arch flattens. Because the transverse arch is part of a triune arch support system, not using it degrades not only the other arches of the foot but also the body as a whole.

Further, absent the clasping motion of the forefoot, we seek stability by over-using our toes. Gripping with the toes can occur with either high, rigid arches or flat, pronated feet. In either case, the forefoot is underactive.

The conventional therapeutic exercise to strengthen this part of the foot is to gather up a towel by repeatedly scrunching up your toes. While doing this strengthens muscles that make the toes curl and grip, it does not activate the deep fascia that creates the forefoot spring. The next practice helps you rehabilitate the coordination of this spring.

---

*From my website healyourposture.com, click on "Resources" and scroll to the course called "Know Your Feet."

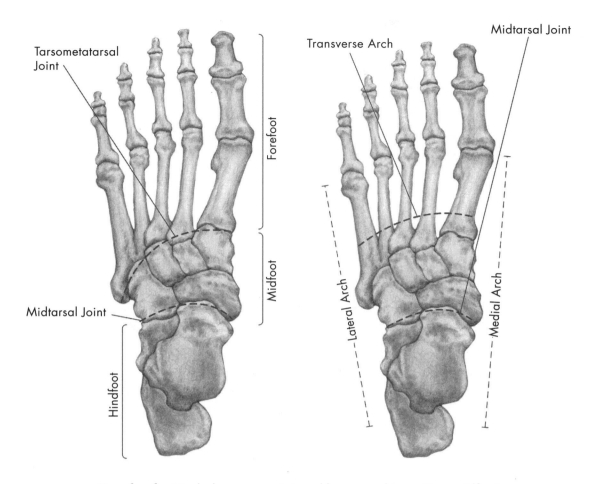

Your forefoot includes your metatarsal bones and toes. Your midfoot includes the bones (tarsals) that are immediately in front of your ankle joint. The midtarsal and tarsometatarsal joints together allow pronation and supination through the transverse arch.

PRACTICE

The Forefoot Dome

🔊 **Practice 34 - The Forefoot Dome Audio and Video**

Sitting in a chair, hinge forward from your hips to bend down and rest the back of your right hand and fingers just above the toes of your right foot. If bending forward this way causes strain, place your foot on a low stool.

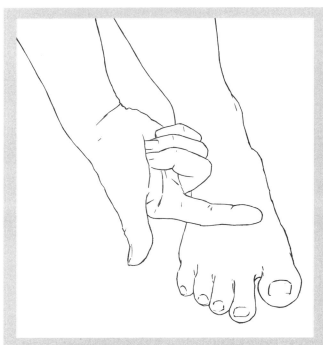

Rest the back of your hand across your forefoot.

If you line up your index finger along the cleavages of your toes, your fourth finger will rest across the tarsometatarsal joint. Now that you've located that joint, move your hand, and lightly place your index finger across it.

Spread your toes wide apart. Picture the whorls on the bottoms of your toes. Those ridges could make toe prints that are as identifiable as your fingerprints.

Now, press down on the floor with the pads of all five toes as if you are making toe prints.

When your toes press down, the underside of your forefoot lifts up to form a shallow dome shape. You will feel a very slight lift under your forefinger and a feeling of activity beneath your arch.

Relax for a few seconds before trying again.

Your toe pads must press straight down onto the floor. They don't scrunch up, and they don't shorten. If you have a habit of clawing with your toes, this will not be easy.

Once more, press down with your toe pads to feel the uplift under your finger.

Then, try to find the doming up sensation in your forefoot without feeling for it with your hand.

Resting between attempts, patiently dome up your right foot two more times. Sustain your last attempt and stand up. You may feel as though a little suction cup has been installed under your forefoot.

> Gently bounce up and down on your right foot, and then compare how the bouncing feels on the other foot.
>
> Before practicing with your left foot, take time to stand and notice any new sensations. Your right foot may feel more alive, or even bigger than before. Your right leg and hip may now feel more stable.

The dome-like action of your forefoot takes place at an acupuncture point known as "bubbling spring."* It might help to imagine a little fountain spurting up under each forefoot as your toes press down.

Your feet may become tired rather quickly doing this practice, the way your tongue gets tired when you're learning a foreign language. You're engaging dormant muscles and sending a new pattern of use to your brain for sensory and motor remapping. Because new movement within your foot must take place in your brain, it's the perceptual aspect of the exercise that makes it effective. Practice it as a sensory meditation rather than as a strengthening routine. Mindless repetition cannot remap your brain's understanding of your feet.

If your transverse arch is underactive, you'll need five-minute practice sessions, two to three times daily. Once you feel clear about the sensation of doming your feet, you can practice anywhere—while taking a shower, for example.

It will not work to try to activate your forefoot while you are walking. The doming action of the forefoot happens much too fast to be ordered by your conscious awareness. By patiently deepening your awareness of this part of your foot over several months, you build the sensorimotor maps that will allow new coordination to emerge on its own. One day you'll notice that your feet feel springier.

Hinge or Catapult?

Ida Rolf taught that the joints between the ends of the metatarsal bones and the tops of the toes formed what she called the "toe hinge." Although this is a useful image for aligning the foot with the joints of the leg above, it's not a good metaphor for healthy foot function. If, in walking, you push off from the toe hinge (the ends of the metatarsals), you're treating the foot as a compression structure. In the biotensegrity model, the forefoot acts as a catapult thanks to the doming action of

---

*The bubbling spring point is connected to the functioning of the kidneys, which according to Chinese medicine, are the body's reservoir of life energy. The new understanding of biotensegrity may echo the findings of the ancient Chinese in acknowledging intricate relationships throughout the body.

the transverse arch. The success of the catapult action in vitalizing gait depends on the tensegral expansion of the body as a whole.

Self-Care for Twenty-First-Century Feet

The following self-massage restores movement to your forefoot and toes. It can help you compensate for the stiffness that results from walking on hard, flat surfaces. You can do it while you're watching TV, or better yet, when you're soaking in the bathtub.

PRACTICE

Self-Care Foot Massage

🔊 **Practice 35 - Self-Care Foot Massage Audio and Video**

Sit with your right leg crossed over your left knee so that you can hold your right foot with both hands. Grasp the middle third of your foot with your right hand. Thread the fingers of your left hand in between the toes of your right foot. Interlacing your toes and fingers can be uncomfortable if your toes and feet are stiff. In that case, rest there for a few moments and breathe.

Try to gently move your toes against your fingers—just a few micromovements. Then rest again.

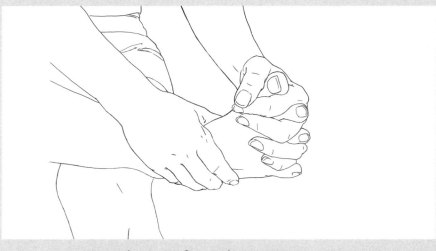

Interlace your fingers between your toes.

From here, use your interlaced fingers to slowly bend and stretch your toes down. And then push them up. Repeat this a few times.

Again, experiment with keeping your fingers passive and wiggling your toes against them.

Now you can introduce movement into the tarsometatarsal joint. Stabilize the middle third of your foot with your right hand. With your left fingers and right toes still interlaced, snugly cup the ball of your foot with your left palm. Your left thumb will wrap over the top of your forefoot. From here, use your left hand to gently twist your forefoot away from your body. Then gently twist toward your body. You are rotating the front third of your foot against the middle third. You are slightly pronating and supinating across the tarsometatarsal joint.

The movement should be extremely slow. If you move quickly, you will not access the deep fascial connections within these joints.

Before repeating the process for your left foot, stand up and feel the result of your efforts. What is your sensory impression of your footing on your right side compared to the left? More pliability? More sole sensitivity? A more vivid mental image of that foot? What effects can you notice elsewhere in your tensegrity body?

Your left foot will now demand equal time.

Aging Feet

Our ability to stand upright depends on a triune balancing system that involves our eyes, the vestibular system of the ears, and the sensory nerve endings in the soles of our feet and ankles.

Humans have become increasingly visually oriented since the development of printed language and reading, and most people unconsciously over-rely on vision to stay upright. At the same time, our feet have lost both resilience and sensory capacity. The relationship between impressions coming from eyes and feet is skewed even in childhood. As we age, the triune balance system degrades further.

Poor balance is one of the reasons elderly people look and feel unstable.

Their heads crane forward as they strain to hang onto the world with increasingly poor visual and auditory systems. Imagine walking around wearing blinders and a noise-canceling headset: you'd need to rely more on your feet to find secure purchase on the ground. But what if your ankles are shaky and your feet are numb?

As we age—and you don't need to be old to be aging—we need to be as conscientious in our care of the feet as we are of our eyes and ears. We notice right away when our eyesight or hearing worsens. But because the feet are not understood to be sensory organs, their contribution to balance is ignored and their problems are addressed with mechanical solutions like orthotics and surgery.

The Digital Age is making many people increasingly reliant on vision, and urbanization has all but deafened our collective feet.

Your developing body consciousness is an investment in your future. How will you look and feel forty years from now?

Seek Uneven Surfaces

The benefits of barefoot walking and running have been in the news since the 1990s, when a study showed that barefoot athletes running on natural terrain had fewer running-related injuries than Western runners sporting high-tech footgear.[3] The sole of a bare foot responds protectively to small pebbles. This involves contraction of deep layers of foot muscles that feet in shoes don't have to make. Because layers of rubber in the shoes mask sensation and eliminate the natural protective behavior of the foot, the shod foot functions with less refinement. It was in the wake of these findings that shoe manufacturers began developing minimalist shoes to replicate the experience of bare feet. But even if your feet and whole body are well toned, resilient, and adaptable, repeated impact of bare feet on pavement is likely to result in injury to feet, knees, hips, or spine.

How, then, can we remobilize our feet and restore their sensory intelligence? Because we've spread pavement over the world, there are no quick answers. Most of us can't relocate our busy lives to a rural setting. But we can seek as many opportunities as possible to walk on uneven ground. One study of people walking barefoot on cobblestones showed significant improvements to balance and mobility, as well as lower blood pressure. Can it be that the perceptual experiences of your feet affect how you manage stress?[4]

I try to give my feet as much variety of angles and textures as I can. During walks, I step on grass or pebbled surfaces in the strips between sidewalk and curb, to offer my feet—and my body as a whole—the micromovements that help keep fascia healthy. I've put a pebble doormat at my kitchen sink and another at my standing desk to knead my bare feet while I work. I fantasize about carpeting my kitchen with stones. Imagine toning your feet while you cook dinner.

REFLECTION
Minimal Shoes

I love wearing my "five finger" barefoot shoes when I hike on mountain trails. The shoes' minimal foot beds let my feet respond to the varying surface of the path, and that invites the rest of my body to adapt and respond. My feet, legs, hips, and spine feel in tune with one another. Of course, it helps that the tall pines urge my midline to join them in praise of the sky.

I love the feeling that each of my toes is independently awake. The shoes make my toe pads want to investigate the ground. When my toes press down onto the ground, activating the inner springs of my arches, I appreciate how delicious it feels to walk.

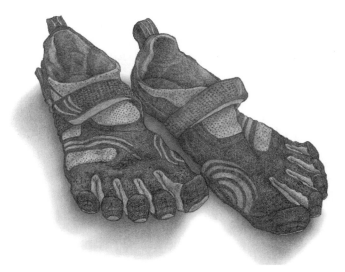

My friend Harmony wears her finger shoes every day and tells me how free it makes her feel. One morning I decide to wear the shoes on my neighborhood walk. Ouch! Going semi-barefoot on concrete feels nothing like walking on a trail. The concrete offers no "give," and the impact of each step jars my lower spine. My feet are incredibly sore after only half an hour and my lower back aches the whole next day.

My experience differs from Harmony's because, being a millennial, she still has fat pads on her soles. Thanks to over seventy years of living on concrete, mine have worn away. So, while there are benefits to wearing minimal footgear, the benefits vary depending on the terrain in which they're worn and on the adaptability of the feet wearing them. I wonder whether my Paleo ancestors suffered from fat pad atrophy. Since they lived only to about the age of thirty, probably not.

Helical Body

When your structure is compressed, walking takes place in a mechanical way, with hips, knees, and ankles operating as hinges and the feet as slabs. But recall that your foot can rotate, propeller-like, around its midline. The midlines of each leg as well as the midline of your body as a whole are axes of rotary motion. Your muscles and fascia are woven around your midlines in something like the basket-weave design of a Chinese finger puzzle. When your posture is open and expanded, the tensional weave offers a spiralic dimension to your gait.

The following two explorations help you feel the subtle counter-rotating tensions that can occur between your feet and spine during walking. They are opportunities to notice the subtle shape-shifting of your tensioned fascia and the "struts" within it. While not meant as lessons in how to walk, you may notice that walking feels smoother after practicing the *Spirals* practices.

PRACTICE

Foot and Spine Spirals I

◀)) Practice 36 - Foot and Spine Spirals I

Stand with your weight comfortably distributed between your feet. Feel your newly awakened toes. Sense the spaces in between your toes. Feel each of your ten toe pads making contact with the ground.

Feel the floor rising up to meet your feet as your body's weight rests down into the floor. Be aware of the space around your body and of your midline deep within it.

Let the movement of your inhalation, and your exhalation, resonate throughout your fascial body—all the way down into your feet.

Now, with minimal muscular effort, make a slightly deeper imprint into the ground with the front third of your right foot and the heel of your left foot. As you do this, your pelvis and lower spine will twist slightly to the left. You may feel your whole body subtly turning leftward.

From there, relax your feet and let your body unwind to neutral.

To clearly feel your body rotating, place your palms together in front of your abdomen as you did in the *Interoceptive Hands* exploration. When you again press down with your right forefoot and left heel, your hands will reflect the rotation of your pelvis.

Now reverse the pattern of your feet, yielding more deeply into your left forefoot and right heel. Feel your fascia responding with a rightward rotation around your midline.

And then relax and unwind.

Continue rotating for a few cycles. Always initiate the rotation with your feet and let your pelvis and chest follow.

If your feet are pliable enough, you will notice that their forward and back alternations are coupled with slight pronation and supination. Do not attempt to make this occur but enjoy it if it does.

PRACTICE

Foot and Spine Spirals II

🔊 Practice 37 - Foot and Spine Spirals II

Keeping your palms together, continue the alternating movement of your feet, as in the previous exercise. This time, keep your heart and head facing forward while still allowing your legs, hips, and pelvis to follow the movement of your feet. This time, your hands will not move.

Press down with your right forefoot and left heel. As your lower spine rotates left, you will sense that your upper spine must rotate slightly to the right so your upper body can continue facing forward. You'll feel this subtle counter-rotation in the area behind your diaphragm. You may even be able to sense the fibers of your diaphragm responding to the rotation.

When you relax your feet, observe the unwinding of your pelvis, and of your spine. If your jaw and face are relaxed, you may even sense release in your thoracic aperture and in your atlanto-occipital joint.

From here, reverse the pattern, pressing down with your left forefoot and right heel, and sensing your pelvis and lower spine rotating to the right. Your upper spine and torso rotate very slightly left in order for your heart to remain facing forward.

Let your arms relax by your sides as you continue alternating the pressures through your feet. Observe the fascial response in your spine.

What is taking place in this practice is a complex orchestration of rotations and counter rotations through many joints besides those of the feet. The movement plays through your knees, hips, pelvic bones, sacroiliac joints, and throughout the spine, including the neck. All of these joints are involved in the movements of healthy walking, as I've described more fully in *The New Rules of Posture.* In the present chapter, my interest is on helping you find a whole-body experience of biotensegrity rather than on identifying the motions of individual joints.

In *Foot and Spine Spirals I,* the micromovements of your feet are translated upward through your fascia to your spine, turning it in the same direction as the feet. In *Foot and Spine Spirals II,* the micromovements of your spine are mediated from above as well as below. The perceptual necessity for the head to face forward in walking activates the counter spiral at the mid spine, as well as a minute counterrotation at the base of the neck.

In areas where you don't easily sense the spiralic flow through your body, two things are likely happening. Fascial adhesions are inhibiting transmission of movement through that area, and your brain has forgotten that movement can occur there. The spiral movement plays through the same diaphragms that you worked with in chapter 5 with *Oscillations II.* Reviewing that practice can help you with this one.

The next two chapters offer a variety of practices that enhance tensegral expansion by decompressing your spine. It will be interesting for you to reconnect with *Foot and Spine Spirals* after spending time with your spine.

REFLECTION
Dog's Feet

My next-door neighbor and I have been sharing our concern about the German shepherd that guards the muffler shop down on the boulevard. When either of us drives past, the dog is always there, pacing the concrete behind a chain-link fence. The doghouse in the yard makes us think he must stay there all night long.

Hazel's voice breaks as she speaks about how this treatment is eroding the pads on the dog's feet. She feels really bad about it. This is a woman who has had four back surgeries and must use a walker to get around. An athlete in her youth, like many people she stopped caring for her body when life got complicated. The irony I notice is that although her own body is now in pieces, she can't help observing what the environment is doing to this poor dog's feet.

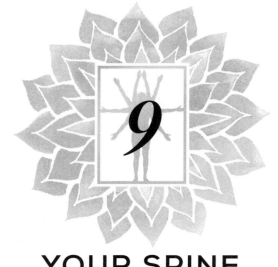

YOUR SPINE
IS NOT A COLUMN

The concept that the spine is a column stems from the mechanical model of the body. In fact, your spine functions like a tensegrity tower—it is more akin to Kenneth Snelson's Needle Tower in Washington, D.C., than it is to the Washington Monument.

Your vertebrae are suspended in your fascial matrix like a string of pearls, not stacked up like blocks. Fascial tissues weave in and around the spinal segments, securing them but also holding them apart. This prevents the vertebral bodies from bearing down upon one another and causing erosion. The "pearls" are more or less mobile, depending on the elasticity of the fascial weaving.

The subtle lengthening of your spine that you feel when you inhale gives you a sense of the labile nature of your spine. If you haven't been able to feel that as yet, this chapter should help.

Evolutionary Journey

In a healthy spine, the vertebrae are configured into shallow forward and back curves. It's a commonly accepted hypothesis that these curves are a product of life's evolutionary journey from sea to land some 450 million years ago. The assumption is that primitive fish moved in the same way as modern fish, with a sideways undulation of their spines.[1] This side bending is a movement your own spine does whenever you reach one hand above your head—to change a light bulb, for example.

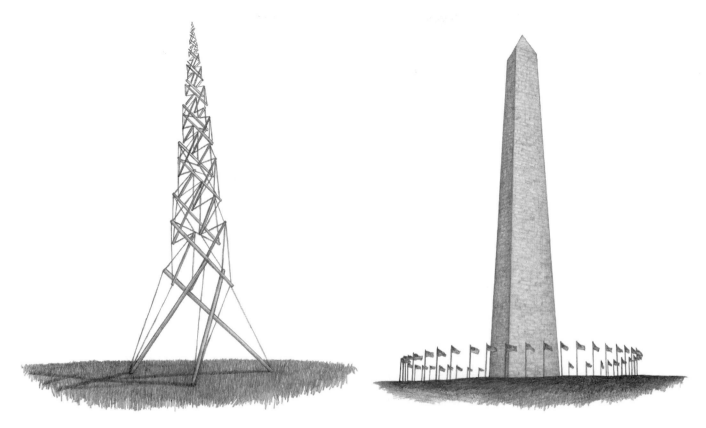

Your spine is more like a tensegrity tower than an obelisk.

When our hypothetical fish first emerged from the oceans, they had to plant their fins into the mud in order to lift their bodies over pebbles and other obstacles. This lifting involved rotating their spines. The combination of sideways undulation with the new axial rotation gave rise to forward and back movements. (You can feel this for yourself: if you bend your torso sideways and then twist, one side of your spine will be subtly flexing and the other side, extending. The more you flex or extend, the farther you will be able to rotate. This is known as **coupled motion of the spine**.)

Over the eons, as creatures ventured into varied terrain, they developed increasingly adaptive structures—limbs and paws to gain better purchase on the ground, hips, and shoulders for additional power. Evolution of a spine capable of **flexion**, extension, and rotation, in addition to side-bending, plus the development of sophisticated limbs, allowed complex movements such as clambering across rocky terrain and swinging through forest canopies. Or belly dancing. Or golf. Or walking.

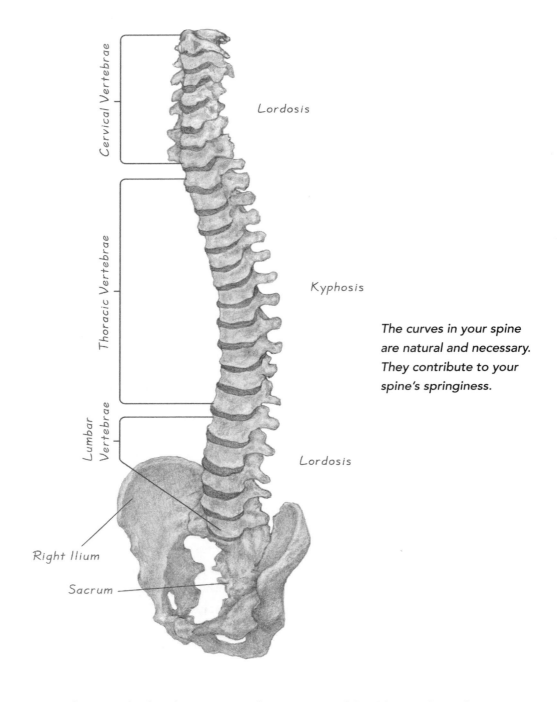

Cervical Vertebrae

Lordosis

Thoracic Vertebrae

Kyphosis

The curves in your spine are natural and necessary. They contribute to your spine's springiness.

Lumbar Vertebrae

Lordosis

Right Ilium

Sacrum

When our bodies have tensional integrity and healthy, resilient fascia, our spines, pelvises, legs, and feet all subtly rotate in order to move us forward. You began experiencing this in the *Foot and Spine Spirals* practice in chapter 8.

Echoing the evolutionary path to uprightness, the individual human spine makes a developmental journey. Before birth, your spine was curved in a "C" shape. When, a few months after birth, you grew strong enough to lift your head, you built the backward curve of the **cervical** or neck vertebrae. By struggling to sit up, you strengthened a second backward curve in the waist or **lumbar** area. The four-legged movements of crawling and creeping were similar to the movements of creatures as they evolved from sea to land. Once standing, the curves in your spine helped absorb the impact of your feet striking the ground.

The spinal curves are normal and necessary. They enable you to move in all three planes. When you flex or extend, you're moving in the sagittal plane. When you twist and turn, you're moving in the horizontal plane. When you rock from side to side, you're moving in the coronal plane. Thus, unlike a fish, you're capable of movement in three dimensions. This adaptability of the human spine lets you function in the field of gravity. Whether you're hiking over mountain scree, playing tennis, or dancing a tango, the relationship between your adaptable spine and your adaptable feet gives your body its sustainability and grace.

Spinal Mobility

If a medical professional applies the terms **kyphosis** or **lordosis** to you, don't worry. These are words used to describe *normal* spinal curvatures. Kyphosis indicates the natural forward curve or slight flexion of your thoracic spine. Lordosis describes the backward curves or slight extension of your neck and lower back. Curves in the spine are problematic only when they're not adaptive—when they can't curve into the opposite direction. For example, a **thoracic** kyphosis that has become encased in stiffened fascia would be unable to extend and rotate. A movement such as reaching for something behind the body—into the back seat of your car, perhaps—could strain the spine. Even more likely, the spinal stiffness would cause the shoulder to overstretch, injuring the shoulder. To prevent that happening again, you'd need to improve the mobility of your spine.

The base of your spine, the triangular-shaped **sacrum**, is moored between twin pelvic bones. Although this makes the pelvis look solid, it is anything but a stable platform. Not only can the pelvis twist within itself, but it is also poised over two round knobs, like ball bearings, at the hip joints. When unrestricted, the hips allow considerable rocking and swaying of the pelvis. This built-in instability of the lower half of your body is what lets you freely move about. Your spine should be adaptable enough to respond to the mobility of your hips, legs, and feet.

Mobilizing the Spine's Foundation

The practice in this chapter contributes to improved mobility between the lower vertebral segments and your sacrum, and between the sacrum, the pelvis, and the hip joints.

You'll start at the base of the spine, heightening awareness of the way the sacrum can articulate with its neighboring pelvic bones, the **ilia**. Through this practice you restore mobility to the pelvis and facilitate greater freedom in your hip joints. You begin to sense the elasticity present within your pelvis, and the fascial connectivity of your pelvis, legs, and spine.

Take plenty of time—weeks rather than days—to explore the sequence of practices in this chapter and the next. Each one offers you improved self-support, adaptability, centeredness, and grace.

Sacred Bone

Your sacrum and ilia rest against one another at the **sacroiliac joints**. The ilia swivel back and forth with every step as shown in the accompanying video. Although the amount of rotation at the sacroiliac joint is tiny, it can make a big difference in the capacity of the pelvis to convey helical motion between the legs and spine while you're walking.

🔊 Practice 38 - Videos of Swiveling Ilia

Your sacroiliac joints are capable of moving back and forth about two to four millimeters. Although this movement is minute, it is essential for fluid motion of the lower back and pelvis. The exploration that follows brings awareness to your sacroiliac joints and encourages normal movement there. The practice is an adaptation of an exercise borrowed from the Feldenkrais Method. Dr. Moshé Feldenkrais, a contemporary of Ida Rolf, founded a gentle and effective system of movement rehabilitation. His approach utilizes brain plasticity through targeted awareness to restore optimal body organization. (For more information, please visit the Feldenkrais website.)

PRACTICE

Preparation for Sacrum Clock

🔊 Practice 39 - Preparation for Sacrum Clock

For *Sacrum Clock* and another practice in chapter 10, you will need to lie on the floor with your knees flexed at right angles and the soles of your feet resting on a wall. If your upper spine is rounded, place a small lift under your neck and head to keep your airway free.

Lie close enough to the wall that your thighs can be vertical. Position your feet hip distance apart. Scoot them upward about an inch, until your toes are resting just above the level of your knees. Spread your toes apart from each other. Let the pad of each toe make contact with the wall.

Positioning your feet may have brought some tension into your legs. Take a moment to relax your calves while keeping mindful contact of your feet with the wall. Let your feet be *touched by* the wall. Imagine vectors that project from the tops of your shins to the ceiling. These imaginary cables will help your legs relax in this position.

Extend your upper arms outward in line with your armpits. Bend your elbows so your forearms are at right angles with your upper arms. Your arms make the shape of a goalpost on a football field.

The backs of your hands rest on the floor. (If your hands don't reach the floor, place folded towels beneath your forearms and hands. The props will make it easier for your shoulders to relax and your chest to expand.)

Allow a slight backward curve or lordosis in your lumbar spine. There will be a tiny puff of air between the floor and your lower back. This is your **neutral lumbar curve.**

Position your head so your eyes gaze straight up at the ceiling. This establishes a neutral curve in your neck. Do not press your neck into the floor to make it straight.

Each time you inhale, feel your upper chest widening—your armpits seem to move apart from each other. When you exhale, let your spine, legs, and head settle ever more deeply into the ground.

As your armpits spread apart from each other, your two elbow points also expand sideways. Each inhalation lengthens the horizontal vector between your elbow points. Gently sustain that expansion as you exhale, and let your head and spine sink deeper into the floor between your elbows.

This breathing practice broadens your back and helps create space for freer movement in your spine.

Sacrum Clock

For this practice, you will imagine a clock face on the front surface of your sacrum. The top of your sacrum is "twelve o'clock." Your coccyx is "six o'clock." The center of the clock is the neutral resting place for your pelvis. When your pelvis is neutral, there will be a slight gap between your lumbar area and the ground. There will also be a sense of spaciousness between your coccyx and your sit bones. Look again at the illustration of the pelvic floor. Your coccyx and sit bones border an area called the posterior or **anal triangle** of the pelvic floor. It is behind your perineal point. Try to keep this area spacious during the upcoming practices.

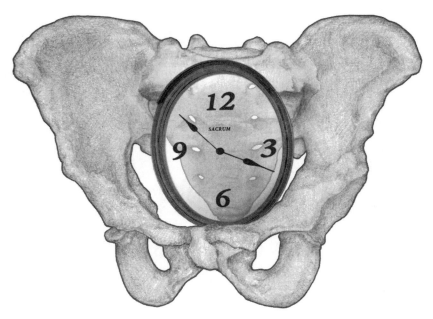

*Imagining a clock face on your sacrum helps you release
and balance your sacroiliac joints.*

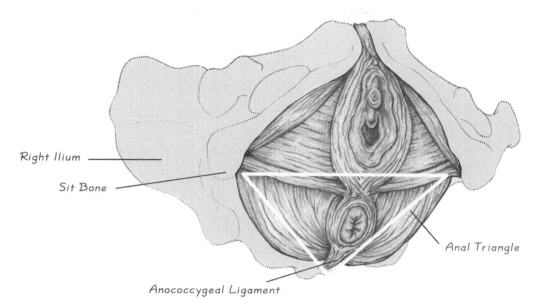

Right Ilium

Sit Bone

Anal Triangle

Anococcygeal Ligament

Spaciousness of the anal triangle of the pelvic floor facilitates the best angle for the sacrum, and thereby contributes support for the spinal curves above.

PRACTICE

Sacrum Clock

◀)) Practice 40 - Sacrum Clock

Lie with your feet on the wall as before, but this time place the palms of your hands on the tops of your thighs just above your groin. Your upper arms will be resting on the floor close to your sides.

Gently press your feet into the wall. As you do this, let your sacrum tip back toward twelve o'clock. Your neutral lumbar curve will flatten a little. Soften your abdomen and imagine your internal organs resting back into your lumbar area as if into a hammock.

Now, relax the pressure of your feet and let your sacrum return to a neutral place, at the center of your clock. Notice whether the anal triangle of your pelvic floor has narrowed. If it has, let your sit bones and coccyx spread apart, melting the tension there. Visualize the tiny strand of fascia between your anus and coccyx becoming longer.

Slightly increase the pressure of your feet against the wall and picture your sit bones staying wide apart. Keep your anal triangle spacious as you repeat the tipping movement of your sacrum.

And again return to neutral.

As you press your feet once more and rest back into twelve o'clock, you will notice that the shift of weight through your pelvis has made your thighbones move up, taking your hands with them. Your thighs have actually shifted forward in the hip sockets.

Your hands will ride down when you return to neutral. Notice how your thighbones then settle back into their sockets. Perhaps one hip settles in more easily than the other. Observe that without wishing for symmetry right now.

From there, continue rolling down beyond neutral into six o'clock. This creates a small arch in your lower back. Your upper back and shoulders continue yielding to the floor. Notice that your thighs now sink even more deeply into your hip sockets.

Once again return to the center of your clock. Pause to soften any tension in your calves, thighs, or pelvic floor.

Softly, slowly, roll back into twelve o'clock.

Then return through neutral and roll down into six o'clock. And repeat. Feel the movement of your thighs in your hip sockets as your sacrum rocks back and forth. Then rest in neutral. Check to be sure you are breathing steadily and gently.

This is a good place to pause and rest, or to take a break and continue the practice during another session.

From here, lean your clock face toward three o'clock, toward the right side of your pelvis. And then back to neutral. And now lean your clock face gently into nine o'clock. And back to neutral. You may notice that it's easier to yield into nine or into three.

Next time you move into the stiffer side, pause there. Imagine your thighbone on that side sinking more deeply into its hip socket. Picture sand pouring into the base of an hourglass. Exhale. And then return again to neutral.

Check that you are still aware of your feet being in contact with the wall and that your calves are soft.

And now begin a slow-motion rocking between three and nine. The movement is so small that someone watching you would not see it. Appreciate the ease with which you yield into the easier side. Be gentle with your wish for the stiffer side to soften.

Notice that as you rest into three o'clock, the nine o'clock side floats slightly upward, away from the floor. As you yield into nine o'clock, the three o'clock side rises.

As you yield again into three o'clock, your right thigh rests back into the hip socket, and your right buttock softens. As you yield into nine o'clock, your left buttock softens, and your thighbone rests deeper and deeper into the left hip socket.

Return to the center of your clock, with awareness of the neutral curve in your lumbar spine. Feel the spaciousness of the anal triangle of your pelvic floor. Breathe.

To finish, slide your feet up along the wall, straightening your knees. Reach your arms up above your head. Relax your concentration. Let your body move in any way that feels comfortable.

When you're ready, roll to your side and rest in a fetal curl for a moment. Then bring yourself up to standing.

Notice how it feels to be upright. Observe how the weight of your body rests through your ankles and into your feet. Notice your sense of presence in this moment. Notice how the world appears to you from this place in yourself.

When you walk, you may be newly aware of your sacrum. Observe how that awareness affects the way you're moving. Perhaps there's a new ease in the way your legs swing under your body into each next step.

Perhaps there's an unexpected shift in your mood.

Tail Space

Poor posture is most obvious in the carriage of your head and shoulders, but in fact, your pelvis is often the literal seat of the problem. When relationships between the pelvic bones and hips are skewed, everything above and below is affected, as you have been able to feel for yourself in the *Sacrum Clock* practice. The meditation helps you experience your pelvis as a base of operations between your spine and legs.

Tucking the tail under—a habitually backward tilt of the pelvis—provides poor support for the spine, restricts movement at the hip joints, and limits movement of the legs. Although tilting the pelvis back—moving into twelve o'clock, for example— is a normal movement of your pelvis, it is not a healthy place for your pelvis to stay.

Chronic shortening of the myofascia around the anus and the coccyx is one of many reasons for the habit of tucking the tail. Many of us have landed painfully on our coccyxes. We were soaring down the skate path on our rollerblades, and wham! This usually happens when we're having fun. Sitting down becomes a trial for weeks afterward. Guarding the injured area shortens fascia in the posterior triangle of the pelvic floor and embeds new brain mapping of the pelvis.

Many myofascial structures of the pelvic floor and hip joints collaborate in shortening the anal triangle. You can begin to release this area by imagining that the anococcygeal ligament can lengthen. The ligament's location between anus and coccyx makes this easy to picture. The ligament itself may not actually get longer, but the visualization causes structures around it to relax.

Experiment by placing one finger lightly on the tip of your coccyx. If your coccyx has been bent under by a bad landing, you may have to reach your finger forward between your "cheeks." After gently locating the tip of your coccyx you can bring your hand away.

Now, without changing anything else about your posture, draw your tail farther forward toward your anus. You are making the tail-tucking pattern worse on purpose, to feel how your tissues contract and to highlight that sensation. Then release, imagine your "tail space ligament" lengthening and your coccyx moving back away from your anus. The movement is subtle, internal, and should not produce an obvious change in the orientation of your pelvis. But notice how that tiny release of the posterior pelvic floor affects your overall stance—you'll feel securely planted on your feet and upright in your torso. You may even notice an interior lengthening sensation as far upward as your throat.

It will be beneficial to review the clock meditation with this added detail in your awareness. And carry your tail space awareness into the rest of the meditations in the book.

There are many reasons for tensions and imbalances in the pelvic floor—sexual trauma, traumatic childbirth, and lower bowel congestion, to name a few. Any of these can affect the function of your body as a whole—your movement, posture, and peace of mind. It will benefit your Body Mandala practice to seek professional help for such issues.

The Minute Hand

Many people feel stiffer on the "nine" or "three" side of their sacrum clocks, with a stiffer hip joint on the same side. If that is true of you, see whether this pattern correlates to your "preferred leg," the one you stand on first to put on your pants. The lumbar fascia on that side of your lower back is also likely to be thicker than on the other side. This is both the deep fascial patterning of your personal contrapposto (see chapter 7) and a habit of your brain.

Once the basic *Sacrum Clock* practice feels familiar and easy, you may be able to remap your asymmetrical pattern by practicing minute-by-minute circuits around your clock face. Begin at "twelve" and find your way clockwise or counterclockwise around the hours. Yield into each minute, traveling as slowly as a minute hand. You will likely find there are flat places in your circuit even though the clock face is round. You may also notice hesitations—areas where the movement feels discontinuous rather than smooth. These hesitations indicate that your brain is attempting to map new coordination at your sacroiliac joints. Respect the hesitations. Patient practice will smooth them out.

Coach yourself to yield more deeply into the flat or bumpy areas. You can refresh the yielding sensation by reviewing the *Rolling* practice from chapter 1. Also recall the way inhalation creates multidirectional vectors through your body. Use your inhalation to expand your interior space and your exhalation to help you yield. Patient interoception invites stiff and matted fascia to soften so that bony surfaces can decompress.

It does not matter whether you make a perfectly round transit around your clock face. The practice is effective without your having to reach perfection. Stop your practice whenever you begin to feel frustrated. A short period of sincere practice will give you a measure of new coordination, but trying to hurry your body into a new pattern will only create more tension.

Walking Integration

After you stand up, take a walk to notice any effect the *Sacrum Clock* practice has had on your legs, hips, and spine. Simply feel. Don't try to analyze it or make something happen. It's fine if you notice nothing at all at first. Creating new movement maps in your brain takes time and patience.*

Healthy coordination is intrinsic to your biotensegrity structure. Walking biomechanics involves the way the bones that comprise each joint float against one another in the fascial matrix, the way the various muscles add impetus, and how the entire fascial net supports and facilitates each contributing joint action. Actually, every cell in your body is involved in every moment of every step.

---

*In *The New Rules of Posture* and in my video course, *Heal Your Posture,* I simplified the mechanics of walking into incremental joint motions. In *Body Mandala,* my intention is to help you embody your wholeness, rather than to focus on what various parts should be doing while you walk.

Over time, we all acquire habits that obstruct tensegral coordination. *Sacrum Clock* and other practices that follow help you revise those habits. By working with micromovements, you reach the deepest layers of your fascial body and reawaken sensations that your nervous system has forgotten.

Recall from the discussion of neural plasticity in chapter 2 that the brain's relationship to the body is highly changeable. According to psychiatrist and neuroscience writer Norman Doidge, walking generates new brain cells and growth factors that strengthen the neural connections involved in learning a new skill.[2] When we feel our bodies differently, we experience our movement differently, and such newly felt movement *is* a new motor skill.

REFLECTION
A Random Pain

I wake up early with pain in my left knee. It hurts to bear weight on it. It hurts to use the toilet, hurts to feed the cat, so I don't even consider a morning walk. Random pains like this tend to assert themselves the older I get.

Okay, I decide, I'll do some stretches on the floor to get my juices moving. I lie down. Without thinking about it, my feet go up on the wall in position for the clock practice. It's comfortable for them to be there.

The knee pain could be sourced in my pelvis. My sacroiliac joints could be out of alignment and tension resulting from that could irritate nerves that affect the knee. I suspend my shins from their imaginary cables, and slowly travel around my pelvic clock. The movement stutters, especially on the left side, and it takes a while for it to smooth out.

Twenty minutes later I stand up feeling bigger. The knee pain is gone. What has happened? I can't be sure whether my clock meditation has realigned my pelvic bones and relieved an impinged nerve, or whether the pain was a transient event that resolved on its own. What I can say with confidence is that by paying attention to the spaciousness and yielding of my body on the floor, and to the micromovements of my pelvis, I affected the tensegral expansion of my fascial body as a whole. More often than not, a random pain can be modulated by embodied wholeness. Not only physical pain. I remember my argument with Richard (chapter 3)—tuning in to my embodiment transformed that pain as well.

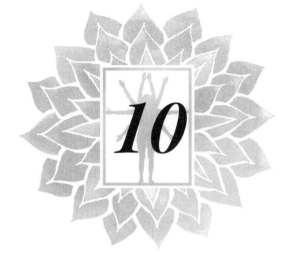

10

TENSEGRITY TOWER

In this chapter, you'll explore your spine as "not a column." By working with vectors projected from your vertebrae into the space behind and in front of your body, you use tensegral expansion to rehabilitate your spine's mobility. This helps decompress your spine and supports expansion of your midline.

Sense Your Vertebrae

Before you begin the next practice, ask a friend to help you feel your individual vertebrae. Tactile contact helps you to visualize the spatial vectors that emanate from your spine and to sense the substance of individual segments.

Sit with your spine in a slight "C" curve. Your partner will "walk" her fingers vertebra by vertebra from hairline to sacrum. The cervical segments are about a finger's width apart and there are seven of them. They may be difficult to locate if you have tight muscles in your neck. Your partner can estimate by counting seven finger widths.

The small projections on the twelve thoracic vertebrae will make them easier for your partner to touch and feel. These are approximately a thumb's distance apart. It's not important to be absolutely accurate—if you miss one or two, it's okay. The idea is to begin to experience your vertebrae as spacers floating in a tension network.

Your partner should proceed slowly enough that you have time to feel the presence of each segment. After counting to twelve for the thoracic segments, count five more for the lumbar vertebrae. These are larger and farther apart. At the bottom, you will feel the flattish triangular spread of your sacrum.

If no one is available to help you with this right now, you'll still benefit from doing the next practice.

One more thing to feel before you begin: reach down to locate a considerable "bump" below your kneecap at the top your shinbone (**tibia**). It's a place you skinned if you were an active kid—remember those scabs? You will project vectors from these points (your **tibial tuberosities**) in the next exercise. I've named them "shin points."

Mobilizing Your Spine

The *Curling into Hammock* practice may initially appear similar to the "bridge pose" performed in yoga and other fitness disciplines. In bridge pose, you elevate your hips and spine in one piece with the goal of raising the pelvis high above the feet. This involves muscular effort in the backs of your thighs, in your "glutes," your abdomen, and along your spine.

In the next practice, your spine curls into a shallow hammock shape rather than making a bridge. By articulating your spine segment by segment, you lengthen the back of your body without shortening the front. In the process, you'll be using your body as a tensegrity system. By doing so, you achieve support through a body-wide sharing of load, rather than by contracting specific muscles.

PRACTICE

Curling into Hammock

🔊 **Practice 41 - Curling into Hammock Audio and Video**

Lie on your back with your thighs vertical, your knees bent, and your feet placed on the wall at a level slightly higher than your knees. Rest your arms in a "goalpost" position and be aware of the multidirectional expansion of your breathing. If this positioning of the arms is uncomfortable, let your arms rest by your sides with your upper arms rotated out and your palms facing up.

Feel the skin on your heels, the balls of your feet, and the pads of your toes being touched by the wall. Relax your calves. Locate the center of your sacral clock and let the weight of your pelvis settle there. Allow a slight space between the back of your waist and the floor—your neutral lumbar curve. Do not flatten your lower spine against the floor.

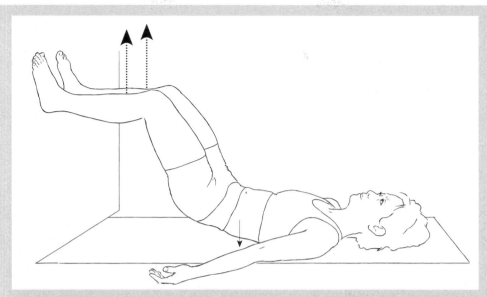

As the vertebrae peel up from the floor, the polarity between the shin points and the individual segments creates a hammock for your abdomen.

Imagine vectors extending from your two shin points straight up to the ceiling. They are like cables holding your legs in place. If there were laser pointers at your shin points, you'd see two red dots on the ceiling.

Now, glide your shin points a few inches upward along those vectors. Your sacrum will rest back into twelve o'clock. Pause there, and be aware of a polar expansion between the top of your sacrum resting down into the ground and the shin points aiming toward the ceiling.

As your shin points rise a little higher, your pelvis begins to peel off the floor. Continue the upward movement, now resting back into your lumbar area. As each successive vertebra yields downward, the segment directly below it peels up from the floor. Each successive vertebra sinks down in opposition to the ascent of your shin points along the imaginary cables.

Avoid pushing your pelvis upward by squeezing your buttocks or tensing the backs of your thighs. Instead, maintain a wide tail space and release the back of your pelvic floor. Renew the strong feeling of polarity between your shin points and the vertebra you are focused on. You are using your tensegral expansion to lift your pelvis. How high it goes is not important.

Continue curling your spine upward, segment by segment, until it seems effortful to go farther. Your stopping place will be unique to you. Let your spine be suspended between the topmost vertebra resting downward and the upward vectors at your shins. Let your abdomen rest back into the hammock of your spine.

From there, slowly unfurl your spine to neutral. You can use your hand on the front of your body to help you visualize the downward vector of each succeeding vertebra. Picture the vertebrae as pearls on a string—you're lowering them pearl-by-pearl. Keep your shin points suspended from the ceiling while each vertebra sinks back.

As you descend, you may find that certain vertebrae are reluctant to yield. Simply notice them for now and continue.

As you pass through your lower back, your lumbar area *will* flatten into the floor. At this moment you may feel a strong engagement of your abdominal core muscles. Appreciate that sensation. Your core muscles engage automatically because of the oppositional expansion between your lumbar vertebrae and your shins.

Continue to roll down through twelve o'clock. When you arrive at the center of your sacral clock, your lumbar segments will rise slightly off the floor, restoring your neutral lumbar curve. Renew the spaciousness in the back of your pelvic floor. Rest there.

To finish, straighten your knees and slide your heels up the wall. Bring your arms overhead for a luxurious stretch of your entire body. Then roll to your side and rest for a moment in a fetal curl.

Find your way to standing and take time to let your spine reorient to your upright posture.

Before the next time you practice *Hammock,* consider whether you had a tendency to contract your buttocks muscles during the roll up. If so, place a small ball, foam yoga block, or rolled-up towel just above and between your knees. Grip it lightly, enough to keep from dropping it. Holding the ball prevents you from overusing your hamstrings and gluteal muscles and helps keep the posterior triangle of your pelvic floor spacious.

Check also that you have a neutral curve in your neck. Your eyes should gaze at the ceiling during the entire cycle. When you curve the lower part of your spine, you may find yourself tucking your chin, flexing your neck, and looking downward. Instead, keep your gaze vertical to sustain your cervical curve.

It's not important how far up your pelvis rises from the floor. What matters is that you experience tensegral expansion. "Walking" your fingers along the front of your body can help you visualize the downward vector of each succeeding vertebra and its polar opposition to your shins. You can do this both on the way up and on the way down.

Notice any region of your spine that resists yielding, or that you don't sense at all. For me, there's an area between my shoulder blades where it's hard to sense individual vertebral segments. I like to spend extra time there, rolling up and down through the stiff area, while keeping my shin points well suspended from the ceiling. I picture each vertebra sinking like a pebble in a pond.

Practice rolling through the vertebrae that resist moving but avoid insisting on immediate release. The source of the restriction may actually lie elsewhere in your body. We will explore some of those places in chapter 11.

Walking with Your Shin Points

After the preceding meditation, you will have developed a clear proprioceptive sense of your shin points. By letting these points lead the swinging motion of your legs, you can add vitality to your gait. As you're walking, picture little headlights on your upper shins. This suggestion will tend to make you land farther forward on each foot—on the entire surface of your heels rather than only on the back edges. You will likely feel more grounded and find yourself pushing off more dynamically from your back foot. To feel this clearly, your spine should be as decompressed as possible. *Curling into Hammock* will have helped but remember also to let your crown point—bregma—rise. Let your peripheral vision encompass the space around you.

Core Coordination and Tensegrity

In the early twenty-first century, core stabilization became an obsession in the fitness community, influenced, in large part, by the 1999 publication of research about the relationship between deep abdominal muscle activation and low back pain.[1] Many people interpreted this research as a call for strengthening of the deep abdominal muscles. What the research actually pointed to was that managing low back pain depended on the precise *timing* of muscle activation rather than on muscle strength. Strength in a particular muscle group does not ensure that those muscles will actually be recruited for daily activities. To date, there has been no definitive research that correlates weak core muscles with low back pain.[2]

Excessive training of abdominal muscles compresses structure and reduces freedom of movement. Watch an old Arnold Schwarzenegger film to see what this looks like.

In the previous exercise, you had the opportunity to experience your core as a spontaneous *event*. I suggested that you likely felt engagement of your abdominal core muscles as you unfurled through the lumbar area. Core activation occurred automatically because of the oppositional expansion between your lumbar vertebrae and your shins—because you were participating in your body's tensegrity. You didn't have to think about recruiting particular muscles. Your nervous system triggered core stabilization because you needed it in that moment.

Core support is a coordinated recruiting of stabilizer muscles as needed, rather than a constant state of abdominal tension. It's an orchestration that occurs throughout your tensegrity system, not a buttressing by specific muscular components.

Stabilization is constantly taking place in multiple areas of your body all the time. Throughout the hammock exercise, various stabilizer muscles in your legs and torso came on line as a consequence of your focus on opposing vectors into ground and space. The muscles you needed were triggered and sequenced, millisecond-by-millisecond. The nuanced movement that evolved out of your vectoring process could not have been accomplished by muscling your body up and down from the floor. When you stood up and walked around later, you may have noticed a subtle shift in how your body felt. Perhaps a body-wide change in your coordination has given you a trace of unaccustomed fluidity.

For that shift to become lasting change in your brain's movement maps, you will need many more exposures to tensegral expansion. Your quiet focus on micro-movements and on vectors activates these maps. Each time you perceive yourself moving differently after a somatic meditation takes you closer to transforming your habitual way of passing through the world.

REFLECTION
A Demoralizing Belt

Although research shows no correlation between core muscle activation and low back pain, my own experience contradicts this. Here's the story.

In *The New Rules of Posture,* I devoted a chapter to the topic of core stabilization. The irony was that when the book came out, I was signing books and teaching workshops while wearing a stabilizing belt a chiropractor had prescribed to control my chronic low back pain. Busted, I decided to heed my own advice. I signed up for Pilates lessons.

Like people I described in the core chapter of *The New Rules,* my abdominals were suffering from amnesia. My experience of my abdomen was a shadowy nothingness. This seemed crazy because I'd been involved in somatic healing for decades. About that time, I found a photo of my college graduation. Slender in my favorite dress, the effect was marred by a protruding belly. Looking back through more old photos, a little paunch was evident as early as age eight.

I believe the Pilates coaching benefited my core by refining my abdominal coordination. Activating my core helped me *inhabit* that place in my body. Within a month the intermittent back pain I'd had for fifteen years was gone. Today, although I don't practice Pilates regularly and my core muscles are probably weak by Pilates standards, I've been free of low back pain for ten years. I'm sure it helps that I've tried to incorporate awareness of vectored movement into all my exercise routines. I try to take advantage of the stabilization offered by tensegrity.

In part 3 of *Body Mandala,* you will have opportunities to apply the fruits of your meditations to large movements that require balance and stability.

Spine Drawers

Every point on or within your body is the potential source of a movement trajectory. In chapter 4, you explored projecting vectors into various directions from your hands. You reached beyond your peripersonal space into the world. You can also reach out from places inside your body, like your heart or your throat.

With respect to the spine, twenty-five vectors extend from the back of each vertebra and the sacrum, radiating into the space behind you like the dorsal fin of a sailfish. In the *Hammock* practice, you opposed your spine's dorsal vectors to the

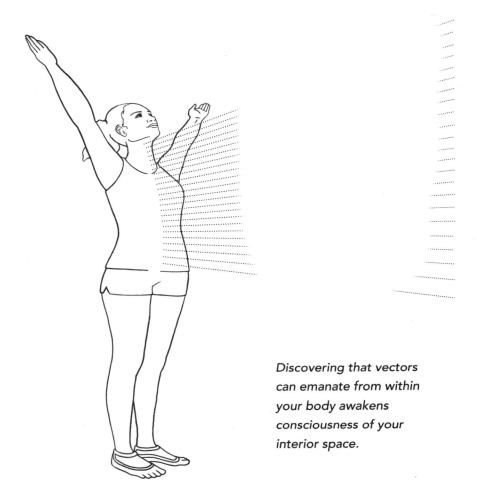

Discovering that vectors can emanate from within your body awakens consciousness of your interior space.

upward direction of your shin points. In the next practice, you work with vectors that emanate from the *front* of each vertebra.

Your spine is deeper front to back than you may have realized. The rounded front surfaces of your vertebrae (vertebral bodies) project forward to approximately one third of your body's depth. The front of your spine abuts your internal organs, which are suspended from it by fascial membranes.

Envision your spine as a tall, narrow chest of drawers. The cabinet has twenty-five drawers, each of which should be able to freely glide out and in (or forward and back). Imagine that the handles for opening the drawers are located on the vertebral bodies. When you inhale, your spinal drawers open. When you exhale, the drawers return to neutral. The opening of a drawer represents its vector—its potential to move forward into the world. When your drawers slide open, your inhalation is accompanied by subtle spinal extension. This movement is so small that it barely affects your natural spinal curves, but not too small for you to perceive it interoceptively.

Like drawers in a cabinet, individual vertebrae can become stuck. Most spines have several segments that have acquired a habit of staying closed. You may have already noticed some immobile places in your spine during the breathing explorations in chapter 6 or during *Hammock* practice. Any "stuck drawers" crimp your posture, compress your midline, and limit your mobility and self-expression. They prevent you from fully opening to the world from that place in yourself.

The animation in this video will help you picture the forward and backward movements of your spine as you inhale and exhale. The movement is tiny but vital for the freedom of your spine.

◀)) Practice 42 - Spine Movement Video

In the *Spine Drawers* practice, you'll observe how your individual vertebrae are involved in the movement of breathing. A light pushing action of your feet makes this more apparent during the first part of the exploration.

At first this practice will seem to emphasize the inhalation phase of breathing. This may tempt you to rush your exhalations. Instead, you need to respect the natural pause that occurs at the end of each outbreath. That pause is the key to optimal functioning of the part of your nervous system that supports relaxation. Restoring your spinal mobility depends on your being relaxed.

PRACTICE

Spine Drawers

◀)) Practice 43 - Spine Drawers

Lie on your back on a padded but firm surface. If your airway feels restricted, place a small lift beneath your head. Have your knees bent at a right angle, with your feet on the floor. Place a thickly folded blanket or firm cushion under the front halves of your feet. Your heels will be on the floor, but the balls of your feet and toes will be on the cushion. The prop maintains a slight flexion in your ankles. This makes your feet feel more grounded than if your soles were flat on the floor. Have your arms and hands in any comfortable position.

Relax on your back for several breathing cycles. Appreciate the natural pause that occurs at the end of each exhalation.

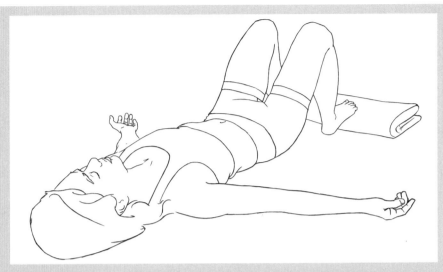

Having your ankles slightly flexed—as they would be if you were
standing—helps your feet feel more grounded than
having them flat on the floor.

Now, while inhaling, press lightly into the prop with the front thirds of your feet. Your heels will feel light, but they don't lift up from the floor.

When you exhale, yield the weight of your heels and ankles into the floor.

Continue like this. When you breathe in, press your forefeet. When you breathe out, yield into your heels.

The pressure of the feet is slight. If you think you're imagining the movement, your pressure is probably just right.

Notice that when your feet press down, your spine extends a little. Your spinal curves don't flatten, but the front of your spine seems to rise. This is the spine's natural movement during inhalation. During exhalation, your spine settles into the floor, and your head rests deeply into the ground. All the little drawers of your spine settle back into their cabinet.

Once again, press your feet and breathe in. Then relax into your heels and breathe out.

From this point on, let your feet relax, but continue to picture the drawers opening as you inhale and closing as you exhale. Spend a few breathing cycles observing where it's easy for you to imagine the drawers opening. Notice where it's hard to picture them responding to your breath.

Now, relax your concentration and return to your ordinary awareness. Stretch and move around in any way that feels good.

Come up to standing and take time to perceive the effects of your meditation.

This would be a good time to review the *Foot and Spine Spirals* practice from chapter 8. There's a good chance that even a tiny bit of improved mobility in your spine and sacrum will have improved your body-wide helical motion. Then, of course, take yourself on a nice, expansive walk.

Acknowledging a Restriction

If you can't feel or imagine a vertebra moving forward when you inhale, that suggests there is compressive tension along the front of your spine, within or behind your viscera. Such tension holds the upper and/or middle spine in a slightly flexed posture. Whether curling in for the heart's protection, or leaning forward into life's intentions or responsibilities, such interior gestures compress the upper vertebrae and prevent your spine drawers from opening. Forward curving of the upper spine drags the head and shoulders forward, contributing to pain and poor posture. It restricts breathing and crimps the wandering pathways of your vagus nerve.

Your sensation of movement and your imagined sensation of movement both occur in your sensory cortex. When vertebral segments are inhibited from moving, your inner gaze—and your imagination—seem blocked. You might not yet be able to sense a vertebra moving forward when you inhale, but if you can clearly visualize it happening, a tendency toward that movement is occurring in your brain. You are revising the brain map for that vertebra.

You can effectively work with a vertebra that has developed a habit of immobility by using a technique known as **focusing**. This method of working with the body's felt sense was developed by philosopher and psychotherapist Eugene Gendlin, Ph.D.[3]

The first step in the focusing process is to become familiar with sensations in front of your stiff vertebra.

You might feel or imagine that place along your spine to have a temperature, a shape, a color, even a sound. Acknowledge your impressions without trying to change them. As you continue meditating on your sensations in this way, they may begin to shift spontaneously. It's important to be sincere in your acknowledgment of the tense area and patient if the tension is too strong to transform right away. Small steps work best. Spend several or many short sessions with this inquiry, rather than attempting to transform yourself all in one go.

All patterns of tension in the body are generated by attempts to stabilize or to protect yourself. If this statement rings true for you, then gratitude is in order. The tense place in your body has been working hard to hold you together. You might consider having a dialogue with your "stuck drawer." Ask it to reveal its purpose for being tense and tight. The following audio offers a short sample of how this might work. Once you have the idea, I suggest doing it without the audio so you can find your natural pace and rhythm and let your own inner dialogue emerge.

Review the previous audio and then move right on to this one. You will still be lying on your back. As always, after completing the exercise, integrate your new sensations into real life by taking a walk. You may notice that the front of your body seems more open than it did previously. Such an effect can occur even if you didn't sense your spine responding during the focusing practice. Your midline may have lengthened anyway. You may notice a sense of opening in your abdominal region, in your heart area, or in your throat. Your voice may sound more resonant. Such effects occur not through posturing with your chest or shoulders but because of your intimate awareness of the front of your spine.

PRACTICE

Focusing

🔊 Practice 44 - Focusing

Bring your awareness inside your body to the place that doesn't seem to move. Lightly rest one hand across your body at the level where you sense an unresponsive vertebra.

The restriction is located inside—in between the stiff vertebra and your palm. Notice your sensations there. Perhaps you feel pressure, tingling, or heat. Perhaps you imagine a color, a shape, or a texture within that space. Perhaps you imagine hearing a low sound or a high sound. Acknowledge your impressions without attempting to change or interpret them.

As you continue being present in this place within your body, you can let your sensations bring an image to mind—perhaps a drawer, a flower bud, a fist. If no visual image occurs to you, simply stay present and curious about your sensations.

Spend the next several breathing cycles focusing on your exhalation and letting your body rest. Invite the vertebra you selected to sink more deeply into the ground each time you breathe out. You are inviting that drawer to exaggerate its restricted pattern. Spend some time with this, looking and listening deeply inside your body. Regard your spine and body with the patience of a loving mentor.

Kindly acknowledge the tension in your spine. Appreciate its effort to support you and to keep you safe.

Listen inwardly for a sensory response to your appreciation. It's okay if your spine doesn't seem to respond right away.

When you are ready, stretch out and move around, relaxing your concentration. Bring yourself to a comfortable seated position. Be aware of the front of your spine as you sit and breathe.

Such opening has potential to activate your parasympathetic nervous system and raise your vagal tone.

A shadow of the original impulse to guard your viscera may still be present.

It's important to respect that. Your healing process involves restoring your relationship to areas of chronic tension in your body. If you try to micromanage the process, you abandon the body schema aspect of your brain where deep change occurs (chapter 3) and instead trigger body image, which can create only an appearance of openness.

The next chapter offers practices that restore ease to areas in your head and neck that commonly tense up under stress. Relaxing your face and throat will bring your spine awareness to fruition.

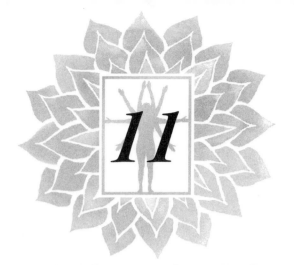

THE LID ON YOUR SPINE

The Digital Age finds many of us living in our heads more than we'd like, and more than is good for our bodies. Getting work done depends increasingly little on physical movement, and more and more on our eyes and on thinking. The emphasis on what's "upstairs" takes a toll on our bodies in countless ways, not least of which is the tension we accumulate in our heads and faces.

Recall that the movement of healthy inhalation involves a mild spinal extension. The practices in chapter 10 helped you notice how tension in the tissues in front of a vertebra can block it from participating in the extension-flexion movements of breathing. This is also true in the neck: tensions in the eyes, jaw, nose, tongue, and throat inhibit the natural micromovements of the cervical vertebrae during respiration. When the cervical vertebrae can't decompress, the neck and head become a "lid" that bears down on the rest of the spine and blocks the natural uplift that your tensegrity affords. This means that the practices you'll do in this chapter will make the practices in chapter 9 and 10 much easier. Releasing the "lid" automatically gives your thoracic vertebrae more space. I wanted you to experience this for yourself. Had I introduced the face practices first, I doubt you would have as clearly perceived the relationship between tensions in your head and body.

Your Jawbone Is Separate from Your Head

The next exploration restores spaciousness and ease to your **temporomandibular joint**. This joint connects your lower jawbone (your mandible) with the temporal

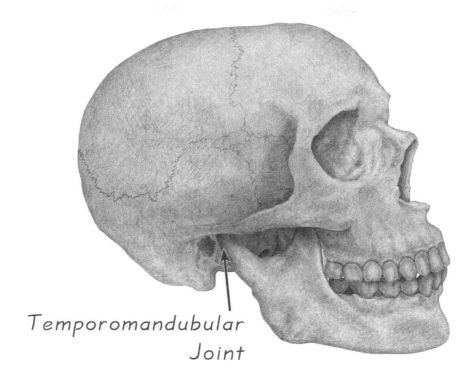

Temporomandubular Joint

bones on the sides of your head. Appreciating the weight of your mandible helps free your face to participate in tensegrity.

PRACTICE

Experience the Weight of Your Mandible

🔊 Practice 45 - Experience the Weight of Your Mandible

Lie on your back with your head resting on a folded blanket. Your legs can be extended or your knees bent with your feet grounded. Have your arms and hands in any comfortable position.

Let your body settle. Each time you exhale, tune into the weight of your sacrum, your cranium, and your spine. Your eyes can be closed or open with a soft focus.

Lift your arms and lightly place your hands against your cheeks. Position the pads of your index fingers just forward of your ears, and your third fingers on your cheekbones. Bend your fourth fingers so their tips rest into the hollows

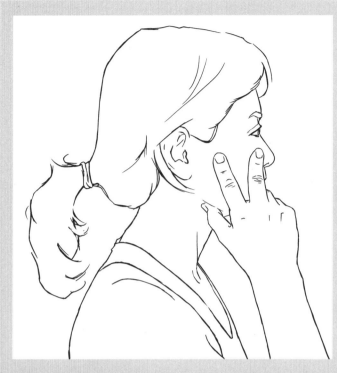

Hand position for heightening sensory awareness of the weight of your mandible.

of your cheeks. Place your thumbs beneath the angle of your jaw. Your thumbs and fourth fingers now hold the widest part of your mandible bone, and your index fingers touch the temporal bones of your skull. Touch lightly.

Gently open and close your mouth, sensing the movement of your temporo-mandibular joint below your index fingers. Now purse your lips together tightly and feel the tissues harden around that joint. You may even notice tension gathering on the sides of your skull and in the back of your neck. When you release the tension in your lips, you will feel your mandible rest back down onto your thumbs. The weight of your head settles more deeply on the ground.

Next, keeping your thumbs beneath the angle of your mandible, relax the other fingers. Then place your index fingers on your cheeks beside your back molar teeth. From there, walk your thumbs and fingers slowly down along the lines of your mandible toward your chin. Take several moments to appreciate the substance and weight of this bone.

Release your hands and rest them comfortably in any position. Feel the weight of your head on the ground.

Now tip your head back as if looking up to see the wall behind you. Lead this movement with your chin. Then, still steering with your chin, bring your head back to a neutral position. When you lead with your chin, your mandible and head move together, as if they were one piece. Notice how this movement feels in your neck.

Relax again, and restore the weight of your head on the blanket. Remind yourself that your head and your mandible are separate. If you like, bring your hands up again to touch your lower jawbone. Try to sense the weight of your mandible as distinct from the weight of your head. It can help to imagine the weight of your lower teeth.

From here, become aware of your upper palate and the "U" shape of your upper teeth. This time, when you tip your head back, lead the movement with your upper palate. And let your mandible lag behind. Let your mandible *follow* the movement of your head.

To return to neutral, draw your upper palate downward. Your mandible follows.

Once more, directing the movement from your upper palate, tilt your head back. You can feel your mandible sliding back toward your ears. When you return to neutral, your upper palate comes down and your mandible floats ever so slightly forward. Appreciate this motion of your temporomandibular joint.

Next, from neutral, turn your head as if looking to your right. Yield the weight of your head toward your right ear. Pause in a comfortable position, even if you didn't turn very far. Sense your mandible resting to that side. Sense the weight of your right cheek, the weight of your right molar teeth. Soften the outer corner of your right eye. Soften the inner corner of your left eye.

Still resting your head deeply into the floor, roll it back to center. And then turn to the left. Sense your mandible and all the features of your face pouring into the left side. Feel weight in your left cheek, weight in your left molars. Sense your eyes resting into the left side of their sockets.

Slowly return to neutral and rest.

Roll onto one side and rest there for a moment. Then bring yourself up to a comfortable standing position. Recall your midline. Sense the movement of your breathing throughout your body all the way down to your feet.

Begin looking around the room. When your face turns to the right, the back of your head moves to the left. When you look to the left, the back of your head goes to the right. Continue looking around, always leading the movement with the back of your head. Your face is a passenger on your head. Your mandible is a passenger on your face.

Be aware of the ground coming up to meet your feet and allow the ground to support your weight. Be conscious of your peripersonal space and of vast spaces beyond it. Recognize these sensations of being present in yourself.

Walking Integration and Expression

If you have room to walk freely, notice the rhythm and the expressiveness of your gait. Freeing up even a portion of the "lid" on your spine can evoke more resilience in your body. Your movement may feel bouncier, more lilting, or more fluid. You may also notice that letting go of your mandible has changed not only your walking rhythm, but also something about your perspective of the world.

It can be interesting to consider a problem—something you've been "chewing on"—from this more relaxed state of mind and body.

The Roof of Your Mouth and Tongue

The roof of your mouth is formed by two mirrored bones called *maxillae*. Shaped like fragments of a chambered mollusk, they form your sinus cavities, the floor of your nose, and part of your eye sockets. Like all bones in your body, your maxillae are embedded in fascial tissue and have the potential to float to an infinitesimal degree. The natural movement of the roof of the mouth is for the maxillae to spread or widen apart from one another when you inhale. Take a moment to feel or to imagine that movement within your oral cavity.

Ideally, your tongue rests softly against the roof of your mouth, barely touching the incisor teeth. Your tongue's presence beneath the maxillae helps support your upper face, provides length for your throat, and tone at the entrance to your intestinal tract. Indeed, your tongue helps align your neck and head.

For most of us, concentrated thought involves verbalization. When you're mulling something over, your tongue and back of your throat (think of the place where swallowing occurs) unconsciously become active, even though you're not speaking. Next time you review your bank statement, notice what's going on in your throat and tongue. Perhaps your tongue is trying to stabilize you against financial ruin.

To begin building a new relationship between your head and neck, try this experiment: widen the back edges of your tongue, spreading it sideways toward your upper back molars. Let your tongue tenderly carpet the roof of your mouth, spreading out to softly touch the inside edges of your upper teeth. There should be no sensation of pressure against your maxillae, only a light, gentle contact.

The tongue's delicate support for your maxillae seems to widen your nasal cavities, making nose breathing easier. It can almost feel as if the air comes directly into your throat without passing through your nostrils. I sometimes call this "nose-less breathing."

You may also notice a sensation of length along your upper throat, as if your head is being released upward. It feels like there's more room within your airway.

If you've learned a different position for your tongue in a yoga or meditation class, remember that those practices are *practices*. What I suggest here is the normal position for the tongue.

Tongue Laxity and Aging

Many of my contemporaries (septuagenarians) have fallen into a habit of forward head posture. One of many causes for this is laxity in the tongue. It is perhaps not coincidental that many of these elders have become mouth breathers.

The *Maxilla/Mandible Breathing* meditation teaches you to release excessive tension in your tongue. But a small amount of tone in your tongue contributes to the uplift in your neck and head.

How you hold your tongue can be a deep-set habit that may have begun with how you suckled as an infant. As you become aware of tension in your tongue—you may be surprised at how pervasive it is. For a while, you'll need to soften your tongue many times a day. Each time, take a nanosecond to register the difference in your breathing and in the easing of your neck.

PRACTICE

Maxillae/Mandible Breathing Meditation

🔊 Practice 46 - Maxillae-Mandible Breathing Meditation

Sit on a bench or stool with the weight of your torso resting just forward of your sit bones. Feel yourself being supported by the flesh of your upper thighs and by the contact of your feet with the ground.

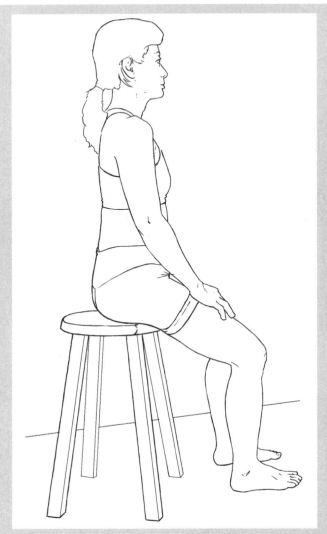

With your weight resting forward of your sit bones, your spine is lifted and aligned.

Recall your midline.

Notice how it feels to breathe through your nose in your usual way. Notice whether there's a feeling of effort in your nasal passages, as if you have to pull the air inside. Observe the sound of your breathing—perhaps there's a faint sniffing noise during inhalation or hissing during exhalation.

Next, swallow to feel the contraction and release of your throat muscles. At the end of the swallowing movement, you will notice a softening of your throat and tongue.

Swallow again, letting the back of your throat—the space behind your uvula—become soft and wide.

Then let your tongue float up to the roof of your mouth. Let it spread across your upper palate like a soft carpet. The edges of your tongue touch the inside surfaces of your upper teeth with pressure so light you barely feel it. Perhaps you will notice that this slight tone in your tongue contributes to a lengthening of your neck—to a lift of your head.

For contrast, let your tongue rest on the floor of your mouth. Notice how that change affects the sensations in your chest and gut. Notice whether it affects your point of view, your mood.

Then replace your tongue on your upper palate. A nanosecond before your next inhalation, picture your back upper molars spreading apart, widening the roof of your mouth. As you inhale, the back of your tongue also widens, and your breath passes into the back of your throat. Air seems to flow directly into your windpipe, as if it has bypassed your nose.

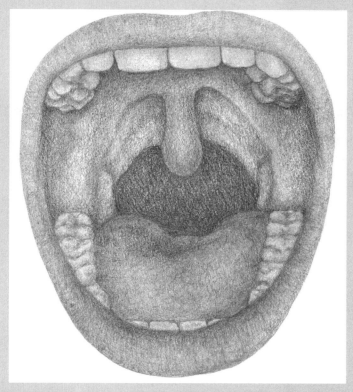

The uvula is a flap of connective tissue located on the same plane as your topmost neck vertebrae. Relaxing tension at that precise location in the back of your throat helps release tension in your neck.

While you are exhaling, bring your attention to the weight of your mandible and to the weight of your lower teeth. Remember the weight of your thighs resting on the chair seat, the weight of your anklebones. Be aware of the space around your body.

Continue, inhaling with a wide, spacious upper palate. When you exhale, feel the weight of your mandible.

Inhalation: soft wide tongue. Exhalation: soft wide throat.

Your breath enters your airway without any effort in your nose. Your inhalation makes no sound.

Because your throat is soft and wide, your exhalation is also silent.

Compare this way of using your nose with the effort of pulling the air through your nostrils. Notice how that sniffing movement narrows your upper palate.

Then return to wide palate breathing.

To finish, be aware of your whole spine moving as you breathe. Picture the drawers in the cabinet of your spine. Observe the drawer that didn't move last time. You may notice greater ease there now.

Integration: Review Your Spine Drawers

At this point, it would be beneficial to return to the *Spine Drawers* practice in chapter 9. With fresh awareness of your face and throat, you may observe that some of the "stuck drawers" feel less restricted than before. Review also the *Sacrum Clock* and *Curling into Hammock* practices. Notice there is greater ease in your lower spine and pelvis when you can soften your "lid."

Eyes in Your Spine

I use two different metaphors for the vectors that extend from the front of the vertebrae—"drawers," which you've already encountered, and "eyes." Eyes open and close just as drawers do. When you look at something, your line of sight is a vector. My students have found that the drawer imagery makes it easier to understand the biomechanical movement of the spine. But the eyes imagery better evokes the experience of opening the front of the spine and being present there. Perhaps you'll dream up metaphors that work better for you.

This section offers two variations of the practices you've already encountered—

they are additional ways to restore vectors to inhibited vertebrae. The audio provides an example of the process. Listen once and then decide how, when, and whether you want to include them in your Body Mandala practice. Once you understand the explorations, practice without the audio. My recorded voice could interfere with your personal rhythm.

PRACTICE

Eyes in Your Spine I

🔊 Practice 47 - Eyes in Your Spine I

Sit on a bench or stool with the weight of your torso resting on your thighs, forward of your sit bones. Be aware of the contact of your feet with the ground and of weight in your anklebones.

Recall your midline. Tune into the ease that relaxing your face has brought to your breathing. Sense how your fascial breathing promotes tensegral expansion throughout your body.

Behind your midline is your spinal cabinet with its twenty-five drawers. Picture the drawers sliding minutely open when you inhale, and receding when you exhale, all without visibly moving your spine. Notice a region where one or several vertebrae do not seem to respond, a section where your interior vision is clouded. Contrast that part of your spine with the places that do respond when you breathe.

Rest your palm on your torso at the level where you sense the immobile vertebrae. Focus inside your body—between your hand and your spine.

Spend the next several breathing cycles appreciating that area *as it is*. The area might seem dark or light, heavy, hollow, dense, or brittle. It could have a different temperature than the rest of your spine. Take time to find your own description.

Then relax your hand and arm.

Experiment with letting that spine drawer (or drawers) recede farther back during your inhalation. You are intentionally exaggerating your dysfunctional breathing habit. The fact that the drawer can close shows *it has the capacity to move*. Appreciate that closing movement during the next several inhalations.

The next step is to imagine the movement reversing. This is a mental action, not something that you must try to do physically. *Just before* you breathe in,

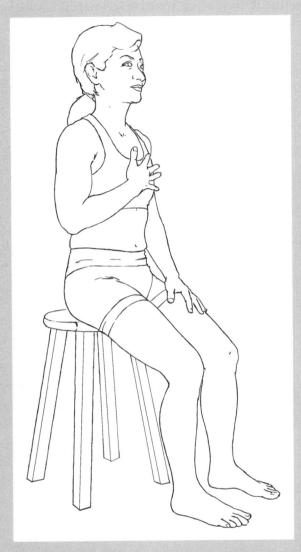

Resting your hand in front of the inhibited vertebrae helps you define the restricted area and appreciate sensations there.

clearly picture the drawer sliding open. After breathing in, relax your focus and let your spine respond. Be willing for it not to respond.

Do this for several breathing cycles and then relax your concentration. Whether or not you feel a response in your chosen vertebra, you now have a clearer sense of its location within your body.

Perhaps it feels a bit more present—like a sleepy eye blinking open.

PRACTICE

Eyes in Your Spine II

🔊 **Practice 48 - Eyes in Your Spine II**

Standing comfortably, renew the ease in your jaw and width in the roof of your mouth. Refresh your awareness of support from the ground.

Locate a place along the front of your spine that feels newly exposed by the previous exploration. Picture an eye opening there. Imagine it looking into the distance from within your spine.

Leading the movement with your spine's eye, turn your torso a few inches to the right, and let your eye gaze into that direction. Continue breathing and notice your sensations as you turn back to center. Notice any tensions in your feet, pelvis, abdomen, or jaw. Notice sensations in front of that vertebra—perhaps a quivering, a tautness, or an ache. Stay with the sensations without trying to interpret or conquer them.

Simply *feel* them.

Leading with your spine's eye, explore turning to the right another time or two. At some point you will receive an internal signal to relax your concentration and return to a neutral state. The signal can be boredom, frustration, physical release, or a quiet voice within you saying, "finish." Listen to your body and rest for the time being.

When you're ready to explore turning your spine's eye to the left, begin without expectation. Your experience of the second side may be different. Recall from the *Peripersonal Space Exploration* in chapter 3 that your spatial orientation can be different on each side. Of course, turning right and left are only two of the myriad potential vectors that can radiate from each one of your spine's many "eyes." Explore any direction that arouses your curiosity.

The *Eyes in Your Spine* practices summon you to reflection and self-study. As you explore deeply held habits, stay focused on the sensations that spontaneously emerge from your body. Should memories arise, resist the mental urge to untangle them right away. Remember that labeling your impressions fixes them in your mind as fact. Instead, linger with your sensory experience. As it fluctuates or changes, stay with the next sensory impression, the next, and the next. You are developing a tolerance for your bodily sensations in present time regardless of their possible linkage to events in your past. Chasing after meaning is like chasing a phantom. Trust your body to share its insight if and when you need it.

Conclude these practices with walking, noticing the quality of your experience when you walk with the new opening along the front of your spine. Tune in to your spinal eyes during your commute or while sitting through a long meeting. For deeper challenge, notice how the eyes in your spine respond when you walk toward another person.

Most of us wish to be open-hearted, to give our vagus nerves full range within our chests. But in fact, it is not always comfortable or safe to stay as open as we feel when we are practicing alone. You can modulate your openness to fit the situation. Opening the heart takes time.

Spinal Decompression

With the next practice we complete the "Deepening" section of this book. The exercise is also a bridge to the "Practicing" section. It's something you can do as a "tensegrity break" in the middle of your busy day. Depending on the formality of your workplace, you can do it right at your workstation.

The exercise borrows from the yoga pose called Cat Cow stretch. The yoga version is done kneeling on all fours and involves a fairly rapid alternation between spinal flexion and extension. You can see a slow-motion version in my video course, *Heal Your Posture.*

What I'm sharing here as "cat meditation" can be done seated or standing.

Because you do it slowly, you have time to incorporate your deepening awareness of your spine.

PRACTICE

Seated Cat Meditation

🔊 **Practice 49 - Seated Cat Meditation Audio and Video**

Sit on a bench or stool that is tall enough that your hip joints are slightly higher than your knees. Your thighs slant downhill. Place your feet about hip distance apart and align your shin points with your second toes.

Sit slightly forward of your sit bones with your weight resting on the tops of your thighs, not back on your buttocks. With your weight distributed this way, the back triangle of your pelvic floor can be spacious, and your coccyx is untucked. Your lumbar spine has a neutral curve. Your perineal point aims straight down to the floor while your bregma point soars upward. Between these points your midline is vibrant. Rest the weight of your leg bones down into your ankles, and feel your feet being touched by the ground. Take a moment to remember that when you touch something, you are also being touched *by* it.

Slightly incline your torso forward over your hip joints, keeping your head in line with your spine. Your gaze will now be diagonally down.

Bring your arms up and place your hands on the wall at the level of your ears and slightly wider than your shoulders. Spread your hands flat onto the wall and imagine you can feel every millimeter of skin being touched by the wall. Pretend the wall is soft, made of velvet.

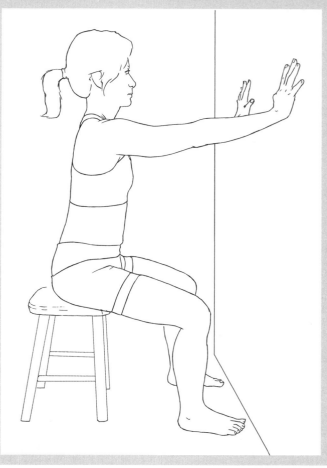

Imagine the wall is covered in velvet and that touching it brings a pleasurable sensation to your palms.

Without moving your hands, draw your elbows in toward your midline and point your elbows straight down toward the floor. When you do this, you will feel your upper arms rotate slightly outward in their sockets and your shoulder blades spread wider across your back.

Your elbows are slightly bent, not locked.

Imagine vectors being drawn down into the floor from your elbows. This subtle action will seem to tug downward on your palms. Your hands don't move, but there's a feeling of traction on your skin. There's also a sensation of activity at the back edge of your armpits.

Lean slightly farther forward, as if you are trying to push the wall away from you. At the same time extend your spine, arching it upward and back to open all of the spinal drawers. Your gaze will now be diagonally up.

From there, imagine the drawers in your neck sliding in and back. Your head begins to nod down and your neck curls forward. Imagine vectors projecting into your back-space from each neck vertebra, like the spines on a sailfish.

Now begin to slide back the drawers between your shoulder blades. This curls your upper spine forward to join the curve of your neck. Below the level of your shoulder blades, your spine remains extended. The vectors of your neck and upper spine reach out into the space behind you, while the vectors of your lower spine and sacrum point forward toward the wall.

Now begin closing the drawers in your middle spine, from the area behind your heart down to your navel. Be aware of vectors reaching into the space behind you from your neck all the way down to your waist.

And finally, slide back the drawers of your lower spine and sacrum. Try to rest your sacrum back without narrowing your pelvic floor.

Pause here with your spine in a C-curve.

Remember to breathe. Bregma is pointing forward into the wall between your hands. Your jaw is relaxed, and your mandible is heavy.

Refresh the awareness of your hands being touched by the wall, your feet being touched by the floor. Picture your shin points aiming forward and your elbow points aiming down. The vectors of your vertebrae fan outward into the space behind you.

Although you are curved forward, the front of your spine feels as long as the back of your spine. You may feel your core muscles working even though you didn't consciously engage them.

From here you will begin to reverse the curves and return to a neutral spine. Start by directing your sacrum forward, bringing twelve o'clock slightly

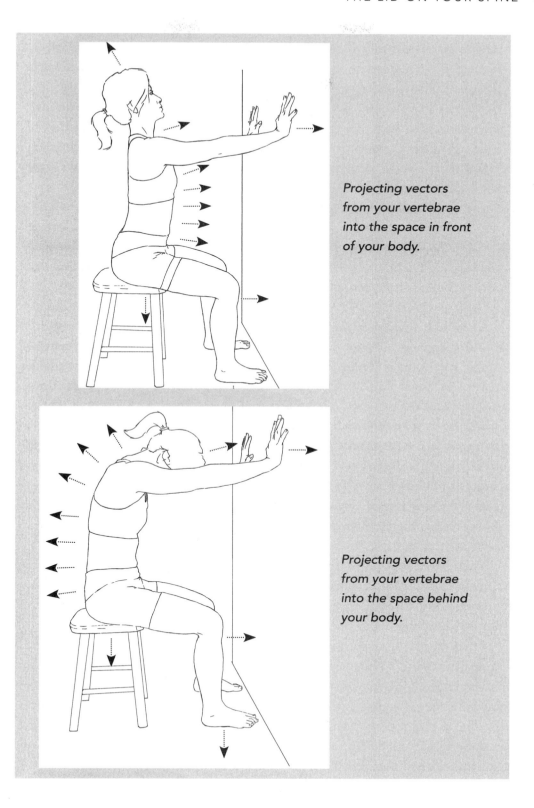

Projecting vectors from your vertebrae into the space in front of your body.

Projecting vectors from your vertebrae into the space behind your body.

forward of six o'clock. Then proceed upward, gliding your lumbar vertebrae forward into a neutral curve. Continue unfurling the vertebrae of your middle back, and then your upper back.

Unfold your neck so slowly that it tests your patience. Keep your head and eyes down and your mandible heavy, while you imagine each neck drawer opening forward. The topmost vertebra is directly behind your uvula. When that one has opened, you can let your maxilla float upward until your eyes are level with the horizon.

In your neutral sitting position, you can sense that the front of your spine, and the back of your spine, are equally long.

When you stand up from this practice, take time to refresh your sense of yielding into the ground, of letting the earth support you from below. Sense the renewed mobility in your spine when you walk.

Seated Cat Meditation incorporates the deepening from chapters 9 through 11 into a single practice. I hope you'll do it often. Here are several details to consider.

The intention is to meditate on your vertebral vectors, regardless of how extended or flexed your spine ends up being. Pause frequently to renew the imagery. The "drawers" or "eyes" are vectors that project from each vertebra into the space in front of your body. The sailfish image represents vectors projecting from each vertebra into the space behind your body. The vectors help you maintain your tensegrity while you fold and unfold your spine. Without them you are likely to revert to familiar movements that buckle your spine, collapsing it at its weak points. Focusing lots of attention on vectors incorporates them into your body schema, remapping your brain and potentially bringing tensegral coordination to everything you do.

The vectors that point down onto the floor from your elbows and into the wall from your hands keep your shoulder girdle expansive enough to make room for new mobility in your upper spine. Imagine your elbow points are laser pointers shining dots of light onto the floor beside your knees.

When you begin curling your neck down from the extended position, part of your spine remains in extension, until, segment-by-segment, drawer-by-drawer, you are flexed into a C-curve. During the transition you will have vectors projecting forward from the lower part of your spine and vectors projecting back from the upper part. The challenge of this meditation is to keep track of your shifting vectors as you flex and extend your spine. Like any meditative practice, it can be tedious at first. With patience and perseverance, it becomes a deeper and richer experience.

By directing vectors from your shin points forward while your feet press down on the floor, you ground the movements of your spine. When you are in the C-curve, your multidirectional vectors activate your core, even though you aren't thinking about your abs. This is biotensegrity in action.

Going slowly when you unfold your neck gives you time to distinguish the sensations of opening through your throat. This subtle opening of the front of the neck replaces the habit of hoisting the head up by overusing muscles on the back of the neck. If you take time to imagine the neck vertebrae opening one by one, your head will reach its destination without your having to forcibly lift it. This is a profound reorganization of your neck. It's helpful to let your eyes gaze downward until you reach the topmost cervical vertebra.

The deep awareness of your spine that you achieve through *Cat Meditation,* along with the previous spine explorations, is of great benefit to your posture, to your awareness of your midline presence and of yourself as a dynamic, upright being. One of the surest signs of aging is an unyielding spine.

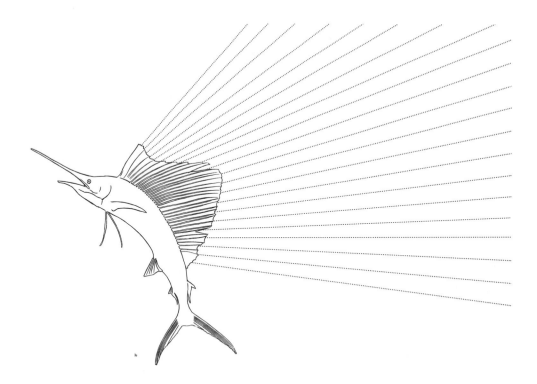

In the Seated Cat meditation, the vectors you project into space from your vertebrae are like vectors from the spines on a sailfish.

Support for Your Midline

I'm aware that the practices in chapters 9 through 11 have been something of a long haul. Most likely you will have embodied some of them more fully than others. You may not need to do the full versions of these practices very often. But a simple practice like *Seated Cat Meditation* can help you renew the basic sensations and benefits of tensegral expansion.

The contemplations concerned with freeing your spine are at the heart of my Body Mandala message. I assume that you now have a deeper somatic understanding of your midline than you did when it was first introduced in chapter 4. Decompressing your spine—restoring its mobility—gives you better support for your midline.

Whether you regard your midline as a symbolic or as an energetic expression of your aliveness, being able to freely access it contributes to your sense of centeredness and presence.

Part 3 offers ways to use your daily activities and your fitness routines as opportunities to practice embodied presence.

REFLECTION

Doubt

I stand at the edge of a chasm, my midline shrinking. If this inner momentum persists, I will reverse my life process, revert to molecules, to atoms. Dread is draining me.

Today I will begin to write the conclusion of this book.

What if there's no audience for my body delvings? What if they're not practical for anyone but myself? Such is my writer's terror.

Standing in my living room, I try to settle my tumbling thoughts and wait for a hint of guidance from my body. I look out the window to the upper limbs of my oak tree. A solitary, hopeful bird pecks at the bark. In my peripheral vision I glimpse my own image in a mirror on the wall to my left. Behind me is a rainy tree-lined country road, a watercolor heirloom that has hung above every fireplace of my life.

I close my eyes. My breath swells the edges of my body, spreading me into the room. I expand. I settle. The wood floor creaks a bit. I'm aware of the slight sway of my uprightness over the knobs of my ankles. Momentarily, I am a tree.

My inhalations push against some sticky drawers behind my heart. But there's no immediate situation to confront—no need to buttress my heart. Can I give it more space?

No. Not yet.

At the base of my throat, there's a lump I hadn't noticed. I swell and settle, letting all of it be there—the lump, the breath, and the ground. Breath stutters. I wait.

My heart thaws a little—warming up and squirming. My collarbones spread out from my sternum and my elbows relax. My fingers uncurl. And my jaw—its clenching, so covert, I hadn't noticed until it melted.

I stand and breathe, knowing I am as safe as anyone can be in a jittery world.

I can dare, for now, to feel what it's like to open my heart and my voice.

PART 3

Practicing

By now, I hope to have convinced you that your posture is a multi-faceted affair. Posture is more than your alignment and balance; it includes what you sense within your body and perceive outside your body. It's your habitual ways of moving and your self-expression—the movements, perceptions, and balancing acts of your daily journey—the ups and the downs.

Self-study through the lens of your Body Mandala helps you make good choices about how you use your body. And mandala practice helps regulate your state of mind by bringing you, again and again, into the present moment.

In the following chapters, I suggest ways to weave your body awareness into your physical conditioning, and into household and work routines.

But first, let's review where you've been so far.

Review

Chapter 1 introduced you to fascia, the Cinderella tissue now being avidly studied by research scientists. The newly discovered neural intelligence of fascia—its capacity for proprioception and interoception—suggests that it is your organ of embodiment. It is largely through your fascia that you experience your body as a whole, and this contributes to your sense of being wholly present.

The main event in chapter 2 was the experience of yielding into contact with the ground. You distinguished between the sensation of yielding and the sensation of collapsing.

This experience helped you understand relaxation as something you accomplish within yourself by learning, as the poet Rilke wrote, to "patiently trust (your) heaviness."

In chapters 3 and 4, you noticed that perception of the space around your body has a supportive effect. You experienced movement as the projection of vectors into the space around your body and felt how your spatial orientation can affect your expression of ordinary gestures. You were also introduced to the potency of your midline as a bipolar vector that organizes your stance and sustains your sense of presence.

In part one, I suggested that you appreciate your bodily sensations without quickly linking them to problems or emotions. I proposed that to expand somatic experience, it's helpful to forgo language for a time. Brain plasticity gives us freedom to change our physical experience and self-expression, but cognitive thinking can get in the way of somatic change. Instead, you can revise your movement maps by becoming curious about your sensory awareness.

Chapters 5 and 6 were devoted to deepening your interoception through micromovements and breathing meditations. You also saw how your vagus nerve contributes to interoception, and thereby to the downregulation of stress in your body and the upregulation of positive emotions and optimism.

In chapter 7, you saw that the classical model of bodily alignment, as a compressive balancing of weights in response to gravitation, is not the whole story of posture. An alternative model suggests that bodies are organized independently of gravity through counterbalancing tensions. The compression model of structure and the biotensegrity model both pertain at times, depending on how you are using your body.

In chapters 8 through 11, you explored your feet and spine in the light of these two models. You understood your feet as sensors rather than as inert platforms, and observed their relationship to the movement of your body as a whole. You investigated the association between breathing and spinal decompression and felt how tensegrity facilitates presence by backing up your midline.

Throughout, you repeatedly asked yourself the Body Mandala questions: what do I sense in my body? How do my sensations affect my stance, the way I'm moving, and how I'm seeing the world around me?

Moving Forward

Human bodies are designed to move. Indeed, all living creatures move in order to obtain their food. And the process of *mechano-transduction,* through which our cells convert mechanical stimuli into chemical responses, helps us understand that movement is essential for the nourishment of our tissues. Movement and life seem to be one and the same thing.

Movement and sensation are also inextricably linked. Lack of proprioception makes it almost impossible to move. Conversely, immobility blocks our ability to fully sense ourselves or our surroundings. The practices in this book use movement to boost your sensory literacy.

To integrate your body awareness into daily living, your daily living must include a healthy helping of movement. If you have a fitness discipline, adding yielding and vectoring to what you already do will be easy and will deepen your sense of presence as you work out.

Few of us have abundant free time to spend on slow-paced interoceptive practices. But once you've deepened your body awareness, you can incorporate it into the things you already do. When you're working out, you've already set aside time for your body, so you only need to fold in your deepened awareness. In that way, your fitness routine becomes part of your Body Mandala practice. Your growing somatic literacy also helps you incorporate the mundane movements of daily affairs into your practice of presence.

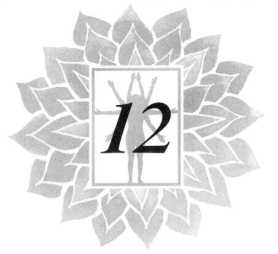

12

EMBODYING TENSEGRITY IN MOTION

To be embodied is to live in harmony with the exquisite intelligence
that resides within our bodies, attuned to the wisdom conveyed through
sensation, and in acknowledgment of the physical conduit of spirit.

Living in the Sagittal Plane

The furious pace of life in the twenty-first century makes equanimity hard to sustain for more than a few minutes at a time. Life rushes full speed ahead while we, sedentary, hang on to our seats and stare fixedly at screens. Our collective focus is sagittal—tunnel-like. Thanks to the internet, we are becoming mentally sagittal as well: we feel entitled to immediate answers and have little patience for research or reflection. Conversational styles take on a laser-like quality as well. Talk show guests drill one another with opinions, calling it a "roundtable discussion."

The more we live in the sagittal plane, the more diminished our spatial orientation becomes. Awareness of people or events outside our immediate focus is vague. Our worldviews contract around the current concern, emotion, or incident. Hyper-focus is a normal response to traumatic events, but constantly being in this state takes a toll on vagal tone, respiration, posture, and social connectedness.

Although it seems specific to the Digital Age, tunneling of awareness has evolved over many centuries. In chapter 1, I suggested that our Paleolithic forebears participated in streams of consciousness in common with everything around them. Not merely aware of the space around them, our ancestors were integrated into their surroundings. We can imagine that they viewed themselves—if they viewed themselves at all—as aspects of the tensional integrity of all life.

During the subsequent Agricultural and Industrial Revolutions, humans progressively narrowed their physical and mental endeavors to interact with tools and machines, harvests and quotas. This narrowing of attention coincided with awareness of a separate self and erased the prehistoric, holistic perspective of aliveness.

Pity our poor twenty-first-century bodies. Our physical and mental endeavors have condensed the world to the dimensions of the screen in front of us. Our tissues grip our midlines, constraining our capacity for spacious body attitudes and generous, multidirectioned gestures. Our tensegral systems solidify into compression structures. Narrowed perceptions become straitjackets that confine our movements to the forward direction. The natural resilience and grace of our bodies is ruined by the fascial adhesion that results from repetitive movements.

Further, hyper-focus on an immediate thing or task seduces us into merging with it. We are individual beings, but whenever we meld with a deadline, an idea, a complaint, a project, or a person, we are not fully present in ourselves.

With your lover or your infant, merging is a good and healthy state. With your computer screen, not so much.

In this chapter, I share a sequence of practices that counteract the sagittal and sedentary tendencies of modern living. I do them every day. Besides being beneficial on their own, they demonstrate how to blend your somatic literacy into the movements of conventional exercise. I offer these practices not as ends in themselves but as templates for finding support and balance through orientation to ground and space.

Distracted Walking

"Distracted walking" has become a new category of injury in the medical community. It refers to preoccupied pedestrians who stare at devices while walking into poles and falling off train platforms or even cliffs.[1]

The Leonardos Practices

I learned the following set of movements from Dr. Phillip Beach, a New Zealand osteopath, acupuncturist, and movement theorist. Dr. Beach named his exercises after Leonardo da Vinci's iconic drawing of *Vitruvian Man*. The practices that follow are my adaptations of Beach's work.

Beach's research examines the primal origins of movement. He proposes that human movement—both the outward activities of the body and the internal movements of organic functioning—derives from the folding and twisting of embryonic tissues. In Beach's model, embryonic movements create energetic fields or pathways from which all human movements evolve. One of these fields winds through the body like counterrotating helices.

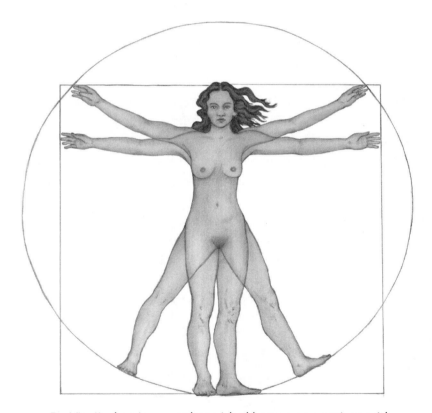

Da Vinci's drawing correlates ideal human proportions with geometry as described by an ancient Roman architect named Vitruvius. The Leos exercises, however, do not seek Vitruvius's geometric ideal but rather reawaken tensegral expansion. The name, Leonardos, helps you remember the start positions for the exercises.

The *Leonardos* practices address the helical field by evoking rotational movement of your hips, pelvis, spine, and shoulders. Because these exercises involve actively loaded whole-body stretching, they both condition the fascia and contribute to your felt sense of wholeness. The rotary motions engage diagonal pathways through the body where fascial tissues are abundant. By integrating rotational movements of the spine and limbs, the *Leos* prime your joints and fascia for the contralateral movements of walking. When you perform them with attention to yielding and to vectors in space, they help develop presence. They're my favorite antidote for sagittal-plane living.

Preparing for Leonardos Practice: Eyes in Your Hands and Feet

The need or desire to touch or grasp something initiates most of your movements. Accordingly, your hands are among the most sensory rich places in your body. Tapping into sensation in your extremities triggers reflexive coordination of your whole body.[2] By bringing awareness to your hands and feet in this (or any other) exercise, you capitalize on that coordinative reflex.

You can boost awareness by imagining "eyes" in your hands and feet. A powerful symbol in many cultures, I'm borrowing it as an ideokinetic suggestion to activate points of sensory perception.

To find the eye in your hand, lightly graze your palm with a finger of your

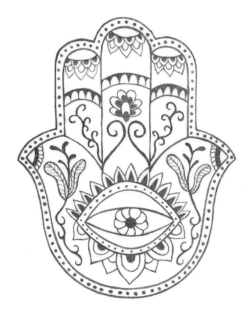

A hand-shaped amulet known as Hamsa is common throughout the Middle East. It has been used as a sign of protection in many cultures throughout history. Most commonly interpreted as a sign of protection, the eye is a powerful symbol of presence.

other hand. Somewhere between the crease lines in your palm, you'll find a spot that is especially sensitive. Designate that spot as your hand's eye. In the upcoming series of exercises, you will be reaching out with the eyes in your palms. I prefer this instruction to the more common directive in yoga classes to stretch out with the fingers. Opening the eyes of your hands invites the experience of presence and aliveness. When your palms feel alive as you reach out, your fingers extend automatically. Without that feeling of aliveness, it's possible to stretch the fingers in a way that deadens the palm. How you experience your hands as you move through the world affects the movement of your whole body.

Your foot's eye is in a corresponding place, slightly in front of your heel. Lightly touch it now to establish its location.

To set up for the exercise, spread a folded blanket or two over a yoga mat. You will also need a couple of objects to use as focal points. These can be furniture legs or plants, or anything already present in your space.

I suggest you watch the videos for *Leonardos I* and *II* before doing the exercise. Then read through the comments that follow the presentation of the practice. With those additional points in mind, you can explore the *Leonardos* along with me, or go at your own pace.

PRACTICE

Leonardo I

🔊 Practice 50 - Leonardo I Audio and Video

Lie on your back with your legs extended straight down. Spread your arms wide, palms above the level of your ears. Rest the backs of your hands on the ground, palms open. Relax into your fascial breathing and let every cell in your body yield into the support of the ground.

Be aware of your body's midline. Lengthen the midlines of your legs and flex your ankles. Reach down into the eyes of your feet and out through the eyes of your palms. Try to reach out and to yield in equal measure.

From here, lift your left foot up and across your body in an arc, reaching it over to the lower right.

At the same time, reach your left hand farther to the upper left, turning your head to look at an object that is beyond your reach. Reach for the object as if you sincerely desire it.

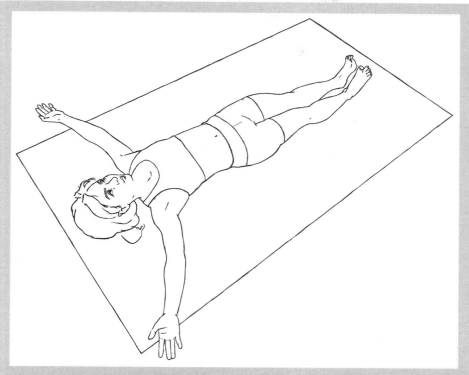

Beginning position for Leonardo I.

Your other limbs are expanded, but the main event is the polarity of the diagonal along your left side.

To return to the starting position, keep your left foot anchored in the space and reach your hand even farther toward your object. Your foot will move a little, but by trying to keep it in place, you will engage the rest of your body in a new way. The reaching action of your arm makes your spine unfold sequentially. It's tensegral movement—everything participating equally.

Let your leg return to the starting position and rest. Notice that your left side now yields more deeply into the ground. Notice the aliveness of the fascia on your left side. Find your own words to describe the difference between your two sides.

Now, arc your right foot up and across your left leg. Reach the eye of your foot over to the lower left. At the same time, slide your right hand out to the upper right, turning your head right to look at an object beyond your reach. With tensegral expansion, your right foot and right hand reach in opposite directions. Imagine your foot pushing down on a pedal. It does not matter whether your foot touches down onto the floor.

To return, keep your right foot anchored in space while you reach your right hand farther toward the object. Even though your hand doesn't go very far, this action makes your spine gradually unfold back into center, segment by segment, from the top down.

Then let your leg return to the starting position.

Do a few moments of *Oscillation* practice before going on to the second exercise. I like to combine *Leonardos I* and *II* before standing up to sense my body and walk around. But this can also be a good place to stop for now.

PRACTICE

Leonardo II

🔊 **Practice 51 - Leonardo II Audio and Video**

This time, separate your legs so your feet are as far apart as is comfortable for you. Flex your ankles and plant your heels firmly on the floor. Bring your arms above your crown and rest your left hand in your right palm. If there were eyes in your armpits, they would be opened to the sky. Feel the expansion through your midline, and simultaneously let your body yield into the ground.

Reach up and across your body with your left hand. At the same time press strongly down and back with your left heel, turning your left leg inward around its midline. These actions roll your torso to the right. Your right hand stays above your crown on the floor.

Enjoy the diagonal polarity between the eye of your left foot and the eye of your left hand. To feel more expansion across the front of your hip, you can reposition your left leg. Your head stays relaxed, yielding to the ground, even though your eyes are reaching for your object.

To return to neutral, keep your eyes and hands reaching along the diagonal while you strongly push your foot down as if it is on a pedal. The action of your leg will untwist your spine from the bottom up.

Rest on your back, and renew your perception of being supported by the ground.

Now put your right hand on top of your left hand. Arc your right arm up and over toward your chosen object while pushing strongly down and back

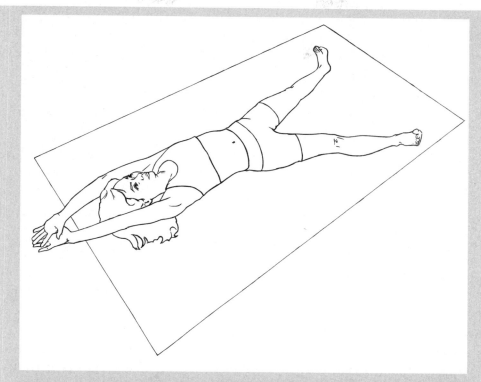

Beginning position for Leonardo II.

into the floor with your right heel and turning your right leg inward. Your hand reaches out while your foot pushes back. Your eyes reach out, but your head yields to the ground.

Continue reaching for your object while you strongly press the eye of your right foot in the opposite direction. The action of your foot will unfold your spine and torso from the bottom up.

Let your spine settle by reviewing the *Curling into Hammock* practice. Even though your feet are on the floor instead of the wall, you can still find the tensegral expansion between your vertebrae and your shin points. Try to roll up one vertebra at a time.

Then slowly unfold your spine.

Bring yourself to sitting, sustaining your sensations of yielding to the ground and expanding into space. This would be a perfect time for an expansive walk.

Once you feel comfortable with the choreography, the *Leonardos* sequence offers a rich menu of sensory experiences.

The rotational movement calls upon the shape-shifting capacity of your biotensegrity system. The opposition between the hands and feet establishes tensegral expansion. Although we don't know exactly how it works, sensory engagement of the hands and feet seems to activate holistic core control. This means that imagining you are actually touching something with your hands and feet contributes to your coordination. Expansive whole-body movement also tunes your fascia.

I sometimes imagine that I'm brachiating through a tree canopy when I do these practices. I imagine my hands reaching for the next branch that I can swing from or for a delicious tree-ripened mango. My feet reach out to clasp the limbs on which I imagine myself poised. Because I am actually resting into the safety of the ground, I can be both relaxed and expansive.

By marrying the sensations of yielding with the action of reaching out, you are practicing active composure. You are teaching yourself to relax and make an effort in equal measure, building that sensorimotor map in your brain. And, with all parts of your body participating, you are also practicing tensegral movement.

If tension in your shoulders limits their range of movement, you will not be able to comfortably roll across your armpits as demonstrated in the video. In that case, you can keep your nonreaching arm resting close to your side. Consider seeking professional help through bodywork or targeted stretching exercises to release your shoulder tension.

Be sure that your eyes accompany the trajectory of your reaching hand. Contemporary life tends to split apart the natural integration of our sensory organs and our movements. Much of contemporary experience is conveyed through digitized media while our bodies are set on autopilot. What we see and hear often bears little relation to what we're doing. This exercise helps bring eyes and body back together. If you perform the exercise without engaging your eyes, you'll notice a difference in the quality of your body's response.

It's important that your ankles be **dorsiflexed** (with your toes drawn up toward your knees). If you do the sequence with your toes pointed like a dancer, you'll notice that although it's a nice stretch, the result is less profound.

When you feel ready, practice the *Leos* without listening to the instructions.

You can then incorporate the body awareness you've gleaned from all the previous practices. Going at your own pace, you can remind yourself to yield into areas you've previously identified as compressed or stiff. You can incorporate awareness of your front spine—the "eyes" or "drawers" along your spine. You can be aware of your peripersonal space even though you are lying on the floor. You can monitor your breathing, keeping it steady, spreading your tongue wide, and breathing through your nose.

For ease in remembering the pattern, here are the basic rules:

- Starting positions are arms apart and legs together, or legs together and arms apart.
- Initiate the movement with the limbs that are together.
- To return to neutral, reach out with the limb that did not initiate the current sequence. The initiating limb then becomes an imaginary space anchor that helps you sequentially unfold your spine—from the top down when you're reaching with your arm; from the bottom up when you're reaching with your leg. Your "anchored" hand or foot will move a bit, but your intention to keep it in place causes you to engage the rest of your body in a novel way.
- Your eyes travel the same trajectory as your reaching hand.

More Leonardos

Leonardos III and IV follow similar patterns of tensegral expansion, except that you begin from a prone (face down) position. You may find them more challenging. It's a good idea to place extra padding on the floor so your breasts will not be uncomfortable when you roll across them.

PRACTICE

Leonardos III and IV

🔊 Practice 52 - Leonardos III and IV Audio and Video

Begin with your arms spread in a wide V and your feet together with ankles flexed. Your toes will be curled up onto the floor.

Keeping your leg straight, reach your right foot toward the ceiling and then arc it behind you to your left, letting your torso rotate. Turn your head right to look at something that is beyond the reach of your hand. Adjust your left leg and foot to rest the outside edge of that foot on the floor. You will feel a strong polar expansion along a diagonal line between your right hand and right foot. At the same time, your head yields to the floor.

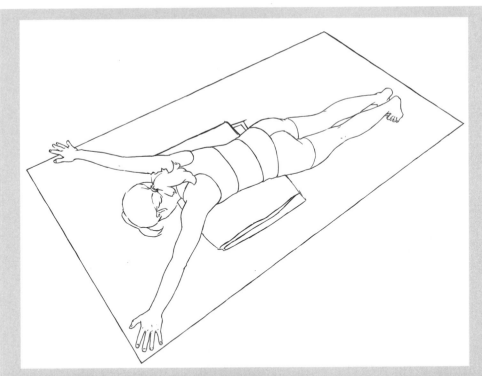

Beginning position for Leonardo III.

To return to your starting position, reach your right palm along the floor as far as possible. Keep an imaginary space anchor on the sole of your right foot. Gradually your leg and spine will be drawn back to the prone starting position.

For the other side, reach your left foot up and then behind you to your right, turning your head to look beyond the reach of your left hand. Keep both ankles flexed. Be sure to adjust the angle of your right leg so the lateral arch of that foot presses against the floor.

For *Leonardo IV*, begin with your legs in a wide V, ankles flexed, and toes curled up. Extend your arms above your crown. Rest your right palm on top of your left hand.

Push down strongly with the toes of your right foot to begin turning your body to the right. As your right shoulder lifts from the ground and your armpit opens toward the ceiling, your right arm sweeps behind you for a delicious diagonal stretch. Keep your ankles flexed. When your legs rotate, you'll be supported by the inside arch of your right foot and the outside arch of your left foot.

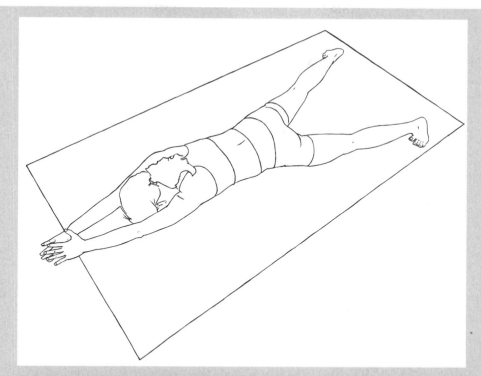

Beginning position for Leonardo IV.

To return, imagine a space anchor on your right hand, and reach your right foot farther down along the diagonal to slowly unwind your body back to the prone position.

Repeat the process on the second side, pushing down with your left toes to rotate your body to the left. Your left armpit opens toward the sky as you sweep your left arm behind you. Turn your head to look beyond your hand. Enjoy the diagonal expansion on the left side of your body.

Return by anchoring your left hand in the space and reaching your left foot farther down along the diagonal.

Once you have returned to the prone position, bring your hands down and push yourself back into *Child's Pose*. Spend several moments breathing into the back of your ribcage.

Pandiculation

Pandiculation is the involuntary whole-body stretching that accompanies transitions between sleeping and waking. When Sensei gets up from a nap, he never fails to do his "downward dog" and "upward dog" yoga poses. Humans, too, stretch and yawn upon awakening. The *Leonardos* are like full-body yawns. Pandiculating movements probably reset the myofascial system in readiness for movement.[3] It's discouraging that cultural conventions prevent most people from publicly pandiculating after sitting through a long meeting or lecture. Imagine a world in which stretching in public spaces was encouraged, a world in which our bodies' need for movement was acknowledged.

Resilient Walking

The high proportion of fascia in our bodies—recall from chapter 1 that humans are similar to kangaroos in this regard—indicates that healthy use of our bodies incorporates springy and bouncing types of movements. Springiness is the manifestation of fascia's capacity for storage and release of kinetic energy.

In the introduction to this book I mentioned that "museum walking," a term coined by James Earls, is tiring because continual stopping and starting relies on muscular control. There's not enough space in a crowded museum for tensegral expansion and fascial energy storage. Consider also "kitchen walking," "grocery store walking," or "small dog walking." These gaits have a halting but monotonous rhythm, devoid of lilt or uplift. They express compression rather than tensegrity. The spine, rather than rotating, stiffens into a pillar, and arms lose their connectivity with legs.

Resilient walking, by contrast, makes use of the multidimensional expansion of your fascial body. The contralateral swinging of arms and legs accompanies a helical motion around your midline. Muscles are engaged, to be sure, but only sufficiently to prime the fascia for rebound and resilience. Unencumbered walking (not carrying anything in your arms) is a rotary activity that involves your whole tensegrity system from foot to crown.

A walking pace that is either very slow or very fast is predominantly muscular. You will make the most of your fascia and invite the spiral dynamics of tensegral motion by walking at a pace that feels moderate and effortless.

Such walking requires space and is best done outdoors, preferably in a natural setting. Being outside invites you to have a panoramic view of the world around you. When you simultaneously open to the space and trust the ground, your perceptions contribute to the tensegral expansion of your body. Your awareness of earth and sky also summons you to the present moment.

Walking on uneven ground whenever possible lets your feet function as sensors rather than as platforms. Stepping on grassy or pebbled surfaces, or on sand, demands that your feet adapt to the minutely varying angles offered by the surface. By association with your feet, your ankles, knees, hips, and spine must also respond to the ground. You will increase your fascial adaptability by using it.

Keeping your perceptual polarity in the background of your awareness, you can incorporate somatic gleanings from earlier chapters. For example:

- Expand your visual perception to include the space to the sides and behind your body. (chapter 3)
- Sense your weight in your malleoli (ankle bones), your rami (pelvic floor bones), and mandible (lower jaw bone). (chapters 2 and 11)
- Let bregma—your crown point—"love the sky." (chapter 4)
- Feel the whole-body response of "fascial breathing." (chapter 6)
- Find the subtle clasping action of your forefoot; feel how it fosters the fascial rebound of your foot and entire body. (chapter 8)
- Soften and open any closed "eyes" along the front of your spine. (chapter 11)
- Swing your "shin points" into each next step. (chapter 10)
- Let your tongue be soft and wide as it rests against your maxilla. (chapter 11)
- Your hands are part of your gait. By sensing your palms moving through the air, you contribute to the coordination of your core. (chapter 12)

I walk several times a week for fifteen to thirty minutes, somewhere between half a mile and two. Some experts recommend walking more than that, but as you may have noticed, expert opinions on health and fitness seem almost as variable as weather predictions. What does seem certain is that a little exercise is much better than none at all. In a Cambridge University study that tracked 330,000 people over twelve years, walking briskly for twenty minutes a day was correlated to a 20 percent to 30 percent reduction in risk of premature death.[4] In the same study, twice as many people died from causes attributed to physical inactivity than to obesity.

In another study, resilient gait was correlated with positive mindset. Negative thoughts caused volunteers to walk with short, shuffling steps, whereas positive thoughts lengthened the amount of time that legs swing freely in walking.[5] Further, walking in nature has been shown to decrease emotional stress, and improve memory, attention span, and creativity.[6] No matter what your age, daily walking is an essential part of your age-defying strategy.

REFLECTION
The Rhythm of the Grass

Trying out some new ultralight walking shoes, I follow my usual custom of stepping on grass or dirt as much as possible. For the first two blocks, though, there's only concrete. The rhythm of my steps feels familiar and ordinary. It has a 4/4-time signature: clop, clop, clop, clop. As soon as I come to a grassy strip, I step onto it. That squared-off rhythm feels awkward now, effortful. I slow down.

I realize that the softer surface allows for a longer downbeat and a rising cadence. Musically it's a triplet: clop-a-da, clop-a-da, clop-a-da. I imagine my fascial body, every cell of myself, yielding into each step. I try to feel that on the inside. My strides are longer now, and there's more articulation in my feet, more of a spiraling action in my pelvis and spine. The triplet meter allows more time for all that movement to take place.

When I step back onto the concrete, my relationship with gravity changes again. The concrete seems to push back at me, increasing the force of the ground against my body. I'm taking shorter, quicker steps, with less feeling in my feet, less movement in my hips, less rotation in my spine. I feel less organic, almost robotic—clop-clop, clop-clop.

By alternating between grass and pavement, I can teach myself to re-create the earthy rhythm even when I'm walking on the pavement. It's not as organic as the real thing, just as practicing salsa in a room by oneself is less satisfying than dancing with a partner. But I can sense more of my body engaged in locomotion. I think it's worth doing.

EMBODYING TENSEGRITY IN STILLNESS

A chair's function is not just to provide a place to sit; it is to provide a medium for self-expression. Chairs are about status, for example. Or signalling something about oneself.

That's why the words chair, seat, and bench have found themselves used to describe high status professions, from academia to Parliament to the law.

EVAN DAVIS, ECONOMIST, JOURNALIST,
AND BBC BROADCASTER

"Someone's been sitting in my chair," growled the Papa bear.

"GOLDILOCKS AND THE THREE BEARS"

Chairless Resting

Our Stone Age cousins' lives were short and brutal by our standards. The necessity to obtain sustenance and shelter and to escape from predators would have made their lives a constant stream of exertion. They walked or ran between three and ten miles a day, in addition to bending, squatting, throwing, lifting, and other movements necessary to survive. Such activities represent the exercise and movement patterns for which our modern bodies are adapted and from which we have drastically diverged.

213

When not killed by predators, our ancestors succumbed to illnesses but most likely did not suffer from deterioration caused by misuse of their bodies.[1]

I picture our forebears as biotensegrities in constant motion, never sitting or standing still long enough for their bodies to become compressed. When not moving, they conserved energy by resting on the ground.

Phillip Beach describes several sitting positions that he calls "archetypal postures of repose," positions he suggests our chairless forebears would have assumed. Modern humans rarely sit on the floor, except in kindergarten classrooms or yoga classes. Both Beach and Katie Bowman,[2] another thought leader in the study of human movement, strongly advise reorganizing our domestic lives to spend more time seated on the floor. Both point out that the activity of getting up from and down to the ground are opportunities to use our bodies according to their genetic heritage.

Having sat on the floor in dance or yoga classes for much of my life, the idea that I should do it domestically wasn't a far stretch for me. Besides, in my seventies, my hip joints aren't as supple as they used to be, and I decided this might help (which it has). I do it most often when watching television, but I've written some of this book from the floor as well, using a low table and my laptop. There are many ways to sit on the floor. Below are examples of floor-sitting styles that I use most often.

Because most twenty-first-century bodies are not adapted to floor sitting, we need props to make them comfortable enough to rest in or to do seated work. I use cushions to make the postures comfortable. I want to be seated in a way that supports my body's capacity for tensegral expansion.

Kneeling

Kneel with your big toes touching and your knees together or apart as is comfortable for you. Sit on your heels. This configuration supports a neutral curve in your lumbar spine, with the "twelve" of your sacral clock slightly forward of "six." Your torso will be uplifted.

If your sit bones rest on the Achilles tendon instead of the heel, your tail is probably curled under and your pelvis tilted back. Your spine curves forward in a "C" shape. To avoid this, slide a pillow or folded blanket into the crease of your knees. The prop will provide support for your pelvic rami and make it easier for you to untuck your tail.

The prop will also help if kneeling puts pressure on your knees.

Seek the feeling of "open eyes" along the front of your spine.

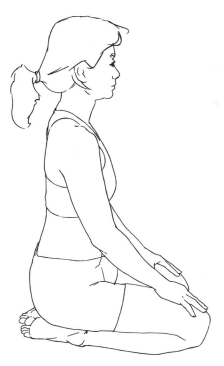

This kneeling posture inclines the pelvis forward just enough to support a neutral curve in the lumbar spine.

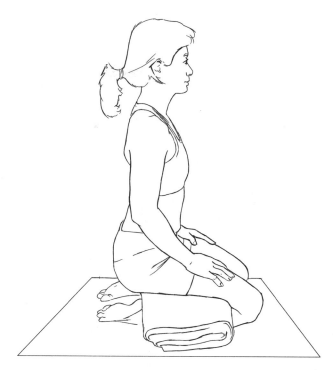

Placing a prop in-between your thighs and calves can relieve pressure on your knees when kneeling and compensate for tight hamstring muscles.

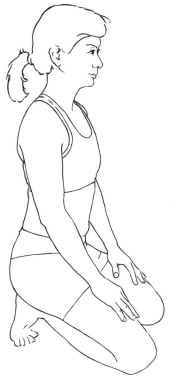

Ease the strain of the kneeling readiness posture on your toes by placing a cushion under your knees.

Kneeling Readiness

If you now tuck your toes under to sit on your heels, you will be in what Philip Beach calls "readiness posture." You are at rest, but because your ankles are dorsi-flexed, you are ready to push off from the ground at any moment. This position is difficult and even painful for many of us because the soles of our feet have stiffened from decades of walking on hard, flat surfaces. You can make the position more tolerable by placing a prop under your knees. That enables you to take advantage of the plantar foot stretch afforded by this posture. But stay within your comfort zone—overdoing this stretch risks injury to the joints between your metatarsals and toes. I sit in this pose only long enough to read an email, or to wait through a TV commercial.

Sidesaddle

You'll recall this posture from chapter 4. You practiced rolling up to it as a way of engaging your midline polarity. For resting in this posture, it's important to distribute your weight equally through both pelvic rami. If your hips are stiff, this

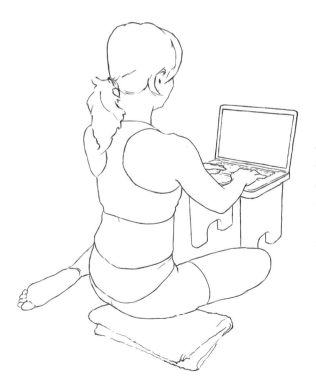

Sitting sidesaddle challenges stiff hips and sacroiliac joints. Sit on a prop to make it comfortable and take it in small doses at first.

won't be comfortable or even possible. The solution is to place a lift under your sit bones. The prop should be high enough that your weight can rest slightly forward of your sit bones, ensuring the neutral lordosis of your lumbar area and inviting length along the front of your spine. Props suitable for floor sitting include bolsters and meditation cushions or a blanket folded to a comfortable height.

Sitting sidesaddle torques your pelvis in a way that is natural but not always comfortable. Most people will find it easier to sit on one side than on the other. This is determined by the habitual pattern of your sacroiliac joints (chapter 9), which affects the tension of muscles and fascia around your hips. Review the *Sacrum Clock* exploration for insight about this. Practice sitting sidesaddle in small doses and work up to spending equal time with your legs resting in the less comfortable direction.

Cross-legs

A small lift under the pelvis facilitates resting in a cross-legged posture. Without a lift almost everyone will roll back and rest behind the sit bones. This causes the front of the spine to buckle, the midline to shorten, and the anal triangle of the pelvic floor to compress. To support spinal extension and spaciousness of your pelvic floor, you need a lift that is high enough that you can feel your weight resting slightly forward of your sit bones.

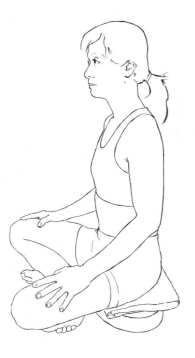

Sit on a prop that positions your hip joints higher than your knees. This allows you to maintain your neutral lumbar curve when sitting cross-legged.

Try to cross your legs at the mid-shins so that your feet are located directly under your knees. This position helps create a stable base, although it also demands flexibility in your hip sockets. Crossing your legs near the ankles is less taxing on the hips but also provides less support. Gradually work up to the mid-shin cross.

Kneeling to Standing

The ability to easily get up and down from the floor is something people under the age of thirty don't think twice about. But once your children are no longer small and the necessity to engage them at their level diminishes, you're likely to spend little time on the floor. Even if you practice floor exercises in a class, you may find it taxing to get up and down. If that rings true for you, take the following exercise to heart. Getting up from the ground is a natural human movement that tones your core and keeps your legs strong and flexible. When it's your turn to be a senior citizen, you'll be glad you've maintained your capacity to get up and down from the ground. It will make you less fearful of the prospect of falling.

In this exercise, you'll move from "readiness kneeling" to standing up. You'll use vectors and spatial awareness to help you coordinate your movement. This means you'll be practicing whole-body tensegral expansion in action. The exercise is also a prototype for how to orchestrate vectors and grounding during exercise disciplines such as yoga, Pilates, dance, and martial arts.

Before reading on, try moving from kneeling on your heels to standing up without using your hands. Notice how much effort it takes and where in your body you feel that effort.

In the video, I demonstrate the exercise in three parts. This is to encourage you to take your time with it if it feels challenging. Be sure part one feels easy before going on to part two.

Kneeling to Standing I

🔊 Practice 53 - Kneeling to Standing I Audio and Video

Start from kneeling readiness posture. Be sure to have ample padding under your knees. Be conscious of your perineal point directed downward, bregma rising up, and the tensegral expansion of your body as a whole. Be aware of your peripersonal space.

In a continuous movement, transfer your weight onto your right knee, simultaneously swinging your left knee forward to plant your foot on the ground in front of you. The first several attempts may feel wobbly on the supporting leg. You might also lift your hip on the side of the moving knee. Try not to do that: swing your left leg directly under your pelvis without lifting your hip.

Use vectors to make this easier. Renew the length of your midline. Then, as

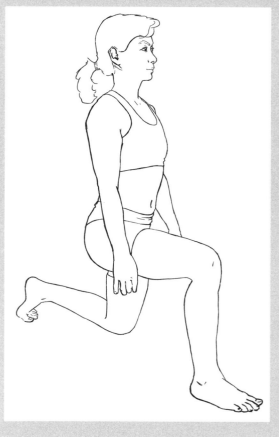

You will pass through this stance on your way from kneeling to standing.

your right toes deepen their contact with the ground, sweep your hands forward and shoot your left shin point forward. Activate the eyes in your hands and look where you are going.

Try it on the other side.

Transferring your weight into your left leg, sweep your right shin point and both hands forward to bring you up to one-leg kneeling.

Depending on the relative strength and coordination of your hip joints, doing this on one side can be much easier than on the other. (This will likely hark back to your "preferred leg" pattern discussed in chapter 7.) To strengthen the weaker hip stabilizer muscles, practice getting up on the difficult side.

An important tip is to quickly **plantar flex** (point the toe) the moving leg. Otherwise you will drag your toes along the floor and lose your balance.

When you feel wobbly, focus on your perceptions of ground and space. That may seem counterintuitive because we've been taught to rely solely on muscular control for balance. To change overreliance on particular muscles entails an important rewiring of your brain maps. In previous chapters, you've been exploring ways in which your orientation to ground and space facilitates tensegral coordination. In this exercise you are teaching yourself to let these perceptions organize a practical movement.

If part one of the exercise is difficult for you, practice by using a piece of furniture to assist you to do the movement. To sweep your right leg forward, hold onto a chair with your right hand. Your left arm will still be free to reach forward and up.

To engage your fascial elasticity, try a slight bounce down into your heels just before sweeping your leg forward.

PRACTICE

Kneeling to Standing II

🔊 **Practice 54 - Kneeling to Standing II Audio and Video**

Begin in the one leg kneeling stance with your right leg forward. Your left knee is under your torso, and your left toes are tucked under. Your left arm can be out to the side for balance or holding on to a chair.

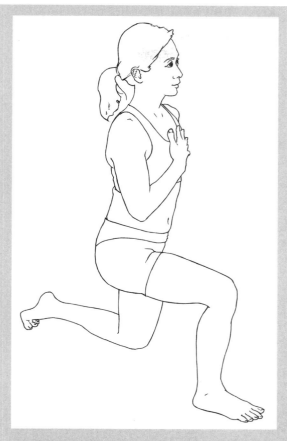

Find a connection between your back foot and your heart.

Place your right hand on your chest in front of your heart. Imagine the fascial connection between the toes of your back leg and your heart. Press back and down with your toes to push your heart forward a little. With this tiny movement you can feel the way your foot can thrust your torso forward. The impulse will seem to travel along the back of your leg and up through the front of your spine. You may feel your gluteal muscles and hamstrings activate when you press your foot. There will also be a stretch along the front of your left hip joint.

Change your position and try this on the other side. One side may feel more smoothly coordinated than the other. Give extra time and extra patience to your less coordinated side.

PRACTICE

Kneeling to Standing III

🔊 **Practice 55 - Kneeling to Standing III Audio and Video**

Start from kneeling readiness. In one continuous movement, transfer your weight to the right and sweep your left knee forward to take weight onto your left foot. You'll be pressing back and down with your right toes to drive your heart forward and up. Sweep your hands forward and up. Let your hands, eyes, and heart all reach forward with enthusiasm.

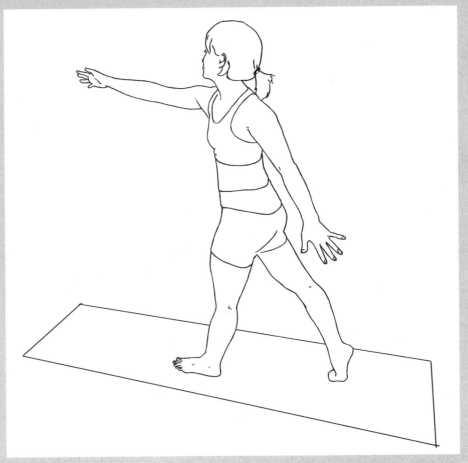

Standing position of this exercise

In the video, I'm using a prop to boost my coordination of the forward sweeping movement. (It's a "swim noodle," but a tray or other object will work as well.) If you imagine that you are offering the object to someone as you stand up, the action feels less abstract than it does when your hands are empty. You'll find yourself getting up more easily. Our brains are wired for practical coordination and for relationship with others.

For greater challenge, sweep your right arm forward with your left leg. You will arrive standing with your left arm back and a slight contralateral rotation in your spine. And vice versa when you practice the other side.

This exercise is a good warm-up before taking a walk. Swinging of the opposite leg and arm demands the same biomechanical responses in the pelvis, hips, and spine as does walking. Don't be surprised if your gait feels freer after practicing *Kneeling to Standing.*

A standard way of analyzing gait is to speak in terms of phases. When you're walking, each leg has a "swing phase," a "stance phase," and a "push-off phase." In the swing phase, your leg flexes slightly at the hip joint, bringing that leg forward of your torso to initiate a step. During the push-off phase, the same hip should extend enough to bring the leg well behind your torso.

Because sitting in conventional chairs flexes our hips to approximately a 90-degree angle, excessive chair sitting shortens the fascia along the front of the hip joints. This compression at the groin limits hip extension during the push-off phase of walking.

By lengthening the myofascia at the front of the hip joint while activating muscles along the back of the hip joint, *Kneeling to Standing* practice counteracts the static hip flexion of chair sitting. The *Leonardos* also help with this.

After working with this exercise for some time, you'll begin to feel a more resilient push-off from your back leg when you walk.

Tyranny of the Chair

According to *U.S. News and World Report,* 86 percent of Americans work at sedentary jobs.[3] Leisure time spent sitting adds up to a startling thirteen hours a day in a chair. Prolonged sitting increases the risk of cancer, diabetes, obesity, and cardiovascular disease. You've probably heard the slogan, "Sitting is the new smoking." Solutions such as standing desks only Band-Aid the deeper issue of the Digital Age lifestyle. My hope and assumption is that humans are smart enough and adaptable enough to find ways to overthrow chair tyranny.

Meanwhile, if you must sit for a living, try doing it with as much tensegrity as possible. Here is brief advice for supported sitting in the workplace:

1. For active sitting situations—times when you are doing work while seated—avoid using the backrest of your chair. Sit toward the forward edge of the seat as if you were on a piano bench. You may have to work up to this if you have a habit of leaning back. Try to use the backrest of your chair only for occasional R and R.

2. Have the seat of the chair at a level that is somewhat higher than your knees. Your thighs should angle downhill. This encourages a slightly forward angle to your pelvis and supports a neutral lumbar curve.

3. Rest your weight into the flesh of your upper thighs rather than on the flesh of your buttocks. This will incline your pelvis slightly forward, and your feet will bear some of your body weight.

4. Another way to think about suggestion three above is to sit slightly forward of your sit bones rather than being poised directly on them. If you alternate between these two options, you'll notice that it's easier to access length along the entire front of your spine when you sit forward of your sit bones. The adjustment is tiny, but it makes a huge difference to the support of your spine and midline.

5. Be conscious of your "tail space"—the distance between the tip of your coccyx and your anus.

6. Sitting with your pelvis inclined slightly forward allows your perineal point to be directed straight downward. If your pelvis rolls back, the perineal vector slants forward.

7. Sitting forward in your pelvis allows you to lean into your work by flexing at your hip joints. That way you "lean in" without losing your tensional integrity. If your pelvis is rolled back, your hips are immobilized, making you bend forward by buckling at the waist or crimping your shoulders or neck.

Refer to chapter 3 in *The New Rules of Posture* for a more detailed discussion of sitting. You'll find a short demonstration of sitting in the *Domestic Bending* video link shared on page 238 of this book.

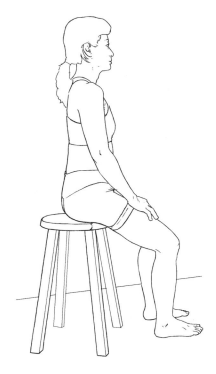

When your thighs slant downward, your pelvic angle can support a neutral lumbar curve.

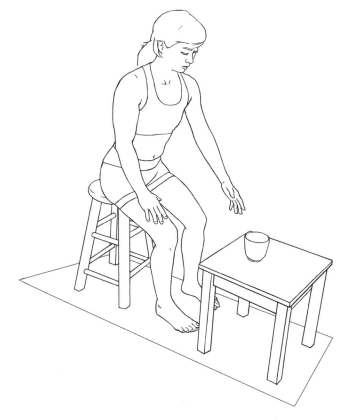

The action of leaning into your work, or bending down to pick something up, takes place in your hip joints.

> **Disc'O'Sit**
>
> Among many props touted to promote correct seated posture, this inflatable cushion is the one I've liked best. When filled with a moderate amount of air, it feels like sitting on a waterbed. The slightly unstable surface makes your pelvis, hips, and lower spine (and by extension, upper spine) undulate slightly while you're sitting.

REFLECTION
Gratitude

For a while, almost all the bodywork sessions I received dealt with the persistent tension on the upper left quadrant of my body. One therapist suggested that the pattern might have originated before I was born, that perhaps I'd been in an odd position within my mother's womb. While this is in the realm of possibility, I've not been inspired to pursue the kind of deep therapy that would be entailed in knowing more. But the suggestion got me thinking about the ways my mother had influenced my life.

Zoe was a schoolteacher from a long line of schoolteachers. "Now, Mary," she'd say, in her teacher voice, and her next words would steer me onto the trajectory of her choice about how to spend my time. Until long after she died, I resented the way she'd tried to shape my experiences to her own taste.

Ida Rolf used to call me "the little schoolteacher," and, not wanting to be anything like my mother, I bristled at the nickname. But I've come to own it. Time changes perspective, and these days I'm grateful to my mother for my "teacher genes" and for so much more.

When I was seven or eight, I used to join her while she did her exercises. We lay on the floor and churned our legs in the air, "bicycling." We poked our heads up and down, trying to prevent middle-age "turkey-neck." Once a week she played badminton, and I went along to watch. She knew, despite her hardscrabble upbringing, that time spent maintaining her body was time well invested. Hanging out with Zoe passed on this belief to me. I also owe her my straight legs. As soon as she noticed that I'd inherited the family knock-knees, she slapped me into ballet classes. And I've been dancing, in one way or another, for seventy years.

Sitting for Men

Friction between the fabric of jeans, an undergarment, and the skin of the scrotum can make well-supported sitting problematic for men. Often these layers adhere to one another like layers of fascia in a body that doesn't move much. To roll forward onto an upright pelvis often requires a manual adjustment men would rather not make in public. This must be why many Western men sit with their pelvises rolled back and their thighs wide apart, the so-called "manspread." Rather than being only an expression of males taking up more than their share of social space, manspread may also be a solution to the chafing, pinching, and poor ventilation of modern trousers.

Historical records suggest that the wearing of trousers evolved in tandem with the domestication of horses. Since our commutes no longer involve sitting astride beasts, perhaps men's attire is ready for a change. I wonder whether rising global temperatures will make garb such as Southeast Asian sarongs acceptable among Western men.

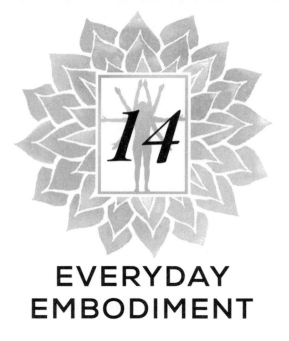

EVERYDAY
EMBODIMENT

Embodied Fitness

Before considering ways to incorporate your fitness routine into your pursuit of somatic presence, let's consider what it means to be fit.

Our ancestors lived as hunter-gatherers for around 84,000 generations. They didn't need to get fit or stay fit. They either were fit, or they didn't survive.

Medicine and technology have made it possible for contemporary humans to survive without being fit, but survival is not the same thing as vibrant, conscious living. An ever-growing body of evidence indicates that an active lifestyle improves your functioning on every level and contributes to healthy longevity. To survive well, we have to move our bodies.

Biomechanist and movement expert Katie Bowman makes a useful distinction between movement and exercise. Her advice is to avoid rote, repetitive exercises, and build your fitness program around the types of movements you can imagine your distant Stone Age cousins doing.[1] This means that a spinning class doesn't qualify—there were no wheels two million years ago. In fact, any repetitive movement in a single line of direction would be eliminated—no more watching TV while running on a treadmill.

Another way of thinking about this is that your fitness program should involve as little time as possible moving in the sagittal plane. Remember that perception and movement are two sides of the same coin, and we already spend too much sagittally oriented time doing sedentary work. Narrowed perception confines movement. We are fascially and biomechanically organized for multidirectional movement and neurologically wired for multidimensional perception. We still have those Stone Age capabilities. We have to recognize the value of reinstating them.

REFLECTION
A Sufi Chant

Being present in yourself, purely and simply, without reference to the success of your personality, or to what you have accomplished in life, is a stage of deepening in all spiritual traditions. A Sufi chant expresses it perfectly: *Men ana? Ana huna.* The question: *Who am I?* The answer: *I am here.* The words mirror the moments of embodied presence emerging through my Body Mandala on my best days.

I'm walking from the kitchen to the dining room with my left arm pressed against my side, fingers curled, clawlike, as if I'd had a stroke. What had I been thinking about?

Oh, of course. I'd been reading a *Time* magazine article about retirement income for single women. Thinking about finances activates my compressive habits every time. But I'm wise to it by now. As soon as I summon awareness of the space behind my body, my anxiety abates. I find ballast in my anklebones. I exhale and my crazy arm yields.

Who am I?

I am here.

There is a cult of strength in the contemporary fitness scene that can make it difficult to incorporate your growing somatic literacy into your workouts. Listening to your own body, perceiving your own needs and limits, can be daunting in an environment of "no pain, no gain."

This environment hinges on the belief that pain is due to weakness, and that muscular strength is a panacea. Understanding of the body's fascial system, once it enters the mainstream, will upend the belief that strength is the primary factor in fitness. Fascia, when properly loaded by the muscular system, is actually stronger than muscle because of its capacity to store energy.

This doesn't mean you should abandon strenuous workouts. Among other benefits, muscular strengthening has an antiaging effect on the brain.[2] But because weight training involves repetitive actions in single planes of movement, weight practice by itself develops compressed bodies. A kettlebell workout is a better option because it combines strength building, flexibility, aerobic activity, resilience, and coordination in multiple planes of action. It also requires engaging your capacity for multidirectional spatial perception.

Your body should feel more open after exercising, not more compressed. You should feel whole, present, and uplifted rather than drained.

Fascial Conditioning

Robert Schleip, Ph.D., one of the founders of the Fascial Research Congresses, has partnered with movement expert Divo G. Muller to develop a program of fascial conditioning. Their objective is to add fascial health to the classical fitness equation of strength, flexibility, and coordination. The Fascial Fitness program includes four categories of training. Knowing about them will help you understand how to care for your "fascial body."

One category is active, whole-body resistance stretches. Unlike conventional stretching routines that target isolated muscle groups, fascial stretches engage long myofascial chains. The *Leonardos,* in chapter 12, are a sample of how such stretches feel. Indulging in full body "yawns" in a variety of twisting or bending body shapes accesses regions of your fascial body that are neglected by your habitual ways of moving. A few bouncing movements or pulsations at the full extent of a stretch stimulates elastic recoil and further awakens your interoceptors.

Using fascia as a sensory organ—being interoceptive—is another category of Schleip's training that overlaps practices offered in *Body Mandala.* Attention to subtle micromovements, such as during the *Oscillations* or *Spinal Drawers* practices, accesses fascial elements sequestered deep within your tissues.

Schleip's third training type involves loading fascial tissues with quick, percussive bouncing movements similarly to what is known as plyometric training. Lightly jumping, hopping, and skipping with your knees only slightly bent activates fascial recoil. The more softly and noiselessly you land—think "cat-like"—the more beneficial the effect. If you deeply bend your knees before jumping or if you land heavily, you engage muscular rather than fascial power. Bouncing on a trampoline doesn't stimulate your fascia because the trampoline absorbs the kinetic energy. You have to find the trampoline-ness *inside* your body.

A twenty- to thirty-minute session of recoil training once or twice a week has been shown to restore the body's elasticity by changing the internal architecture of the fascial webbing.[3] You need to work up to this in graduated stages. If you put too much load on matted, dehydrated fascia, you risk injuring yourself.

Lastly, the Fascial Fitness program includes self-care rehydration massage by using foam rollers in specific ways. Sue Hitzmann's MELT Method offers a similar approach.

In addition, Schleip counsels that fascially directed movement must be varied and multidirectional, rather than repetitive and predictable. Such movement is smooth and elegant and feels effortless and pleasurable. Tensegral expansion is its hallmark.

Whereas gains in muscular strength can be achieved in a few months, Dr. Schleip's research has determined it takes longer to fully reconstitute your fascia—up to two years. So aspiring to fascial fitness is an opportunity to be present with a slow-moving process.[4*]

Self-Cues
for Tensegral Expansion

I use the checklist below when I'm walking, practicing yoga, or working in the garden. The reminders are not in a particular order. You can develop your own Body Mandala checklist with personal priorities depending on the habits you've uncovered.

- Imagine space between the bones in my feet: this invites my feet to relax when I've scrunched them up (usually when I've been trying to avoid doing something).
- Imagine eyes in my palms and soles. Mysteriously, this aids in whole-body expansion.
- Be aware of the back surface of my body from heels to crown, and of the space behind me. "Backspace awareness" is my shortcut to spatial awareness in general. It automatically unkinks my interior web of fascia to some degree.

---

*I included the summary of Schleip's program because it has much to tell us about fitness in general. Unfortunately, as of this writing, there are many more certified Fascial Fitness trainers in Europe than in the United States. A Fascial Fitness DVD is available, however. You can learn about the program by doing a Google search of "fascial fitness today," and you will be directed to the website.

- Tune in to peripheral vision. Find equal value for what's ahead of me and what's in my periphery—this is another way to give myself space.
- Open the "eyes" along my front spine. This is not a set position of the spine, but a feeling that both my spine and my midline are elongated, vibrant, mobile, and comfortable.
- Awareness of the polar expansion of my midline. Whether I'm standing up, folded into Child's pose, or back bending into upward dog pose, there's dynamic polarity between bregma and my perineal point.
- Imagine vectors connecting points on my body to points in the space around me. This is a big help whenever balance is an issue.
- Yield my weight into my bones. This helps me remember that the ground supports me. I have to identify which bones I'm pulling up from the ground when I'm not relaxed:
    - Mandible—it helps to imagine the weight of my lower teeth.
    - Malleoli—draining my weight down into the knobs beside my ankles helps me find my feet and legs when I've lost touch with them.
    - Rami—sitting or standing, feeling weight in these curved branches at the base of the pelvis helps me forego the tendency to tuck my tail under. Diminished tail space immobilizes both my hip joints and my lower spine.
    - Elbows—Feeling the weight of my "funny bones" is an indirect way to invite my shoulders to relax. It helps when I'm driving—or writing a book.
- Fascial breathing. A way to tune in to being whole and present.
- Tensegral expansion—a multidimensional yielding of my skin surface into the surrounding space. It helps me feel that I'm all here. And that I'm big. Big enough for anything that comes.

Yoga and Pilates

Along with walking, yoga and Pilates are my current fitness practices. I attend a weekly yoga class, and most mornings I practice twenty minutes of asana, plus a round of *Leonardos* and *Kneeling to Standing*. Yoga and Pilates are "fascia friendly," but because they don't have a bouncing element, they don't condition fascial elasticity.

Both Iyengar yoga (the style I practice) and Pilates offer ample opportunity to work with the cues listed in the previous section. When you're learning a new coordination—a new asana or Pilates move—it's common for the perception of being supported by the ground to fade away. You may hear an instruction to "ground your feet," yet find it hard to deeply sense your connection with the floor. If your primary way of orienting yourself is spatial, the experience of being grounded remains conceptual rather than being physically felt. Practicing the *Leonardos* can help with this—they teach you how it feels to relax into the floor and make an effort at the same time.

Yoga teachers often use words like "reach," "seek," or "push" to inspire lengthening of the limbs and spine. These instructions become more potent when you picture vectors extending into space from head and tail, shoulder points, elbow points, shin points, hands and feet, and vectors emanating from the front and back of each vertebra. Not all at once though—establish your midline and then add the other polarities one at a time.

Building a virtual tensegrity network *outside* your body expands the spaces *inside* your body. The invisible filaments of your perceptual tensegrity orient your body in space and facilitate your coordination and balance.

Yoga and Pilates both involve proprioceptive awareness. Being precise about body positioning, however, can overpower your interoceptive perceptions. This happens if you listen harder to the instructor than to your own body, or if you become entrained by a competitive atmosphere or by your own competitive nature. Competition destroys your sense of pleasure, increases stress, and by dulling interoception, weakens connection with your fascial body. Your sense of wholeness goes "poof." That's a caveat for both these disciplines, especially if you have a perfectionist bent. Yoga and Pilates both aim for union of body and mind, but we live in a competitive society. A goal-oriented mentality erodes your practice of presence, even in a serene yoga studio.

My own solution to this tendency is to attend to my fascial breathing as sincerely as I can. I try to feel the "whole cloth" of my body, even while I'm focused on details like activating my **transversus abdominus** muscle, or lining up my ankles, knees, and hips. I also remind myself, over and over, to feel the weight of my mandible. Effort generally shows up as jaw tension, and jaw tension makes it impossible to expand upward through the crown of the head.

Managing jaw tension during your somatic practice helps you dismantle it in other areas of life where effort may be concealing itself in your jaw. The fruition of your Body Mandala practice entails bringing what you felt on the Pilates or yoga mat out of the studio and into your car, kitchen, and workstation.

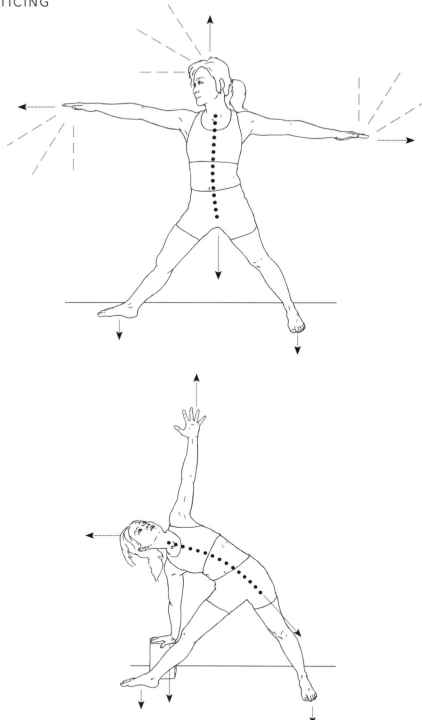

*Vectored movement reshapes your tensegrity as you move
from one yoga asana to another. Your muscles and bones
conform to this higher ordering.*

Cycling and Running

Recalling numerous fifty-mile rides with pleasure, I understand the appeal of cycling. Bike travel is like no other—slow enough to let you smell the passing scenery and challenging enough to make a peanut butter sandwich by the side of the road taste like manna.

Cycling for sport is a different matter. Repetitive motion in the sagittal plane and muscular effort exclusively in the legs and hips mean that cycling erodes fascial health. There's no opportunity for elastic recoil and little possibility for tensegral expansion.

Cycling instigates compressed posture in a number of ways. To avoid pressure into the genital area, bicycle seats enforce a rolled-back position of the pelvis that reduces the neutral lumbar curve and narrows the back of the pelvic floor. The design of racing bikes makes you flex your torso to control the handlebars.

But you must lift your head to see the road. Your midline is buckled at the waist and crimped at the neck. Over time, this position compresses posture and prevents any fluid movement other than cycling. Because their training diminishes the natural rotary capacity of the spine, serious cyclists acquire a characteristic lurching gait. In chapter 7, I suggested that we live ourselves into the shapes we most often assume—or into shapes we assume most vigorously.

If cycling is your favorite workout, consider some additional expressive outlets. Schedule time for exercise that opens and lengthens your body, and that counteracts repetitive movement with varied and unpredictable moves in a variety of directions. Study a martial art or a Latin style of dancing.

Like cycling, running tends to overtrain your body in the sagittal plane. The repetitiveness of running can also diminish body awareness. Unlike cycling, however, there are ways to run that can be beneficial to both your fascia and your presence.

Schleip and others suggest alternating running with short walking intervals. Intense running dehydrates tissues, while walking lets them plump back up with fluid. Schleip further suggests that by running like a gazelle—spending more time in the air than on the ground—runners can take advantage of their fascial elasticity. Incorporating fascial recoil into your running style makes it lighter and more elegant.

Author Christopher McDougall makes the case that humans are natural endurance runners.[5] They outran their prey for nearly two million years before figuring out how to make spears. But they did not run on hard, flat surfaces in foot-coverings that buffered sensations from the ground. Running barefoot on uneven ground, the way our ancestors ran, stimulates proprioceptors in the feet and throughout the body, helping keep you present as you run. By varying your movements—sometimes running sideways or even backward—you might imitate the kind of moves necessary to corner prey. And you give your workout a hint of playfulness.

Domestic Movements

Awareness dims when we do the same thing over and over, and the repetitiveness of domestic activities invites disembodiment. But humdrum moments can be turned into Body Mandala opportunities. You can make domestic tasks into anchor points for revising habits and building deeper awareness, better posture, and likely as not, better moods.

Many domestic tasks involve bending over from a standing position—washing dishes, chopping kale, brushing your teeth, folding laundry, putting on your pants—the list is endless. Any of these tasks can be performed with tensegral expansion, or as a maneuvering of body parts.

Bending or leaning forward into a task happens over and over throughout your day. Take an honest look at how you do it. Where in your body does your bending take place? Do you buckle at your waist? Do your shoulders collapse forward? What about your legs: do your knees lock? Do you tuck your tail? Are your hip joints involved in the action of bending forward?

In the next section you will turn bending over into moments of tensegrity and presence.

Domestic Bending

Refer back to *Curling into Hammock* and *Seated Cat Meditation* to remind yourself of how your body feels when all the segments of your spine participate equally in folding and unfolding movements. In those practices, the front of your spine feels as long as the back. Nothing buckles because there are no weak links and because your entire body participates in the movement.

The purpose of the next practice is to blend the sensation of tensegral folding with the ordinary action of bending over at a sink (or desk, car trunk, mailbox, and so on.)

Bending forward to most domestic surfaces involves curving your spine forward from the pelvis upward. When you're standing at the stove or sink, you need the floor of your pelvis to provide a spacious foundation for your spine. If your pelvis rolls back and your tail tucks under, the pelvic foundation narrows.

Recall that leaning forward into your work from a seated position (chapter 13) necessitates slight flexion at your hips. The same is true when you're standing up. If your pelvis is tucked under, your spine will buckle at the waist instead of folding tensegrally. Hip flexion requires a spacious pelvic floor.

Keeping your knees a little slack—not locked—will make it easier to release your hips and to maintain a spacious "tail space" between your sit bones and coccyx and between your coccyx and your anus. When you bend from your hip joints, you can sustain your neutral lumbar lordosis, the most stable configuration for your lower back vertebrae.

Spaciousness in the pelvic floor also ensures that movement of the spine is supported by your feet. When you tuck your coccyx under, the knees and hips tend to lock. This means that the legs become compression structures, divorced from the body above and unable to participate in tensegral expansion.

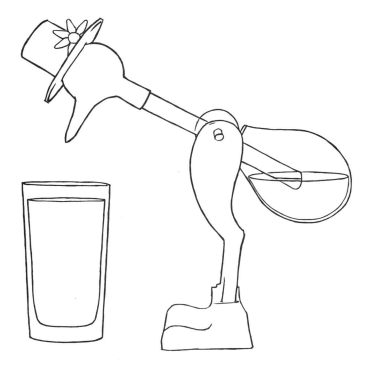

Imagine your own hip joints operating like those of a drinking bird. But let your knees be more relaxed than his.

PRACTICE

Domestic Bending

🔊 **Practice 56 - Domestic Bending Audio and Video**

Sit on a chair or bench tall enough that the seat is higher than your knees. Rest your weight into the flesh of your upper thighs rather than on the flesh of your buttocks. Rest in front of your sit bones rather than directly on them.

Renew your spatial awareness to the front, side, back, above, and below your body. Make yourself big, filling out your skin surface.

Feel weight in your anklebones and in your pelvic rami.

From here, keeping your sit bones wide and your midline elongated, make a small forward-tipping movement. Lean your torso forward. To come back up, push down into your feet. Do this several times to sense this movement taking place in your hip sockets.

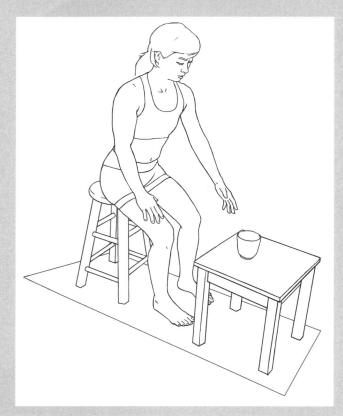

The forward-tipping movement

Next you're going cultivate the same hip action when you're standing up.

Find your perceptual tensegrity in a standing position. Rediscover the weight in your anklebones and rami. Let your sit bones spread slightly apart from one another, widening the triangular space between your sit bones and coccyx. Notice that doing this gives your spine more lift.

From here, try the forward-tipping movement. Perhaps you've seen a drinking bird toy that dips forward like this. Sense the movement that is taking place in your hips.

For contrast, lock your knees and tuck your tail down and do the dipping movement again. With your pelvis in lockdown, you can't do the movement from your hips. Instead, you will bend at the waist.

Return to your neutral stance, with a spacious pelvic floor.

From here, lean your torso farther forward from your hips, keeping your spine elongated. Let your arms drop down as if washing your hands. For many tasks, you do not need to curve your whole spine downward. You can simply slant forward with your midline elongated. Because your lumbar area has a neutral curve, your back does not tire.

When you return to standing, feel your weight yielding down into your rami and feet.

This time, tip your torso forward over your hips and curve your upper body farther down. Your spine can fold forward like it does in the *Seated Cat Meditation*, without buckling in any one place. The front surface of your body is long, even though it is concave.

Now, experiment with bending forward while you lift one leg. This is the action of putting on your pants. Instead of crunching up and tucking your tail, you can use vectors to get support from the space around you. Establish a polarity between your shin points and your coccyx as you slant forward to put your foot through the pants leg.

It will be easiest to balance on your preferred leg—be sure to practice on the other side.

Once you have the knack of bending and straightening tensegrally, you'll notice that the movement feels comfortable and easy. The muscular effort required to straighten up is minimal because your whole body participates in the action. When you bend over from a compressed posture, you have to work harder to straighten out the buckling and crimping of your torso. Repeated bending and straightening from a base of compression tires you out.

You'll be taking up more space when you move this way, so watch your head when you reach into the trunk of your car for the groceries. Reaching into the backseat of a car for a fussy toddler will be more of a challenge. By practicing the movements you can do solo, you'll gradually learn to move tensegrally in relation to real-time events. Cultivating tensegrity throughout your day adds up to many minutes of whole-body presence.

Shoulders

Because my focus has been to elucidate the importance of wholeness and midline, I've scarcely mentioned shoulders in this book. (You'll find a more thorough discussion of the shoulders in *The New Rules of Posture*.) I trust you will have observed that when the front of your spine and neck are elongated and open, your shoulder blades tend to settle onto the back of your rib cage without much coaxing.

Your shoulder joint is the crossroads of your upper arm, your shoulder blade, and your collarbone. The shoulder blade mediates between the arm and the spine, stabilizing and modulating arm actions. The collarbones mediate between the arms and chest. Your shoulders are inherently unstable, but that very instability grants you an extensive range of movement for your gestures of work and play, welcoming and protecting.

Many people believe that good posture necessitates positioning the shoulder blades in a particular way. This makes little sense because if your shoulders are held in place, it immediately becomes impossible to do anything practical, or anything expressive with your arms. Try hugging someone, for example, with your "shoulders back."

Habitual shoulder tension is often a means of compensating for poor support elsewhere in the body. If your feet are unstable or your hips are stiff, your shoulder blades will tend to lift, as if they're trying to help keep you upright. If your upper spine curls in or your head juts forward, your shoulder blades either ride along with the spine, or pull back to counterbalance it. In either case, your arms and shoulders lose their stable connection to your torso. Instead, your fascia accommodates by splinting your imbalanced extremities in place. This prevents adaptable and expansive arm movement.

If your shoulders are particularly stiff, you may need bodywork to restore normal motion. Targeted stretches can also help. You can find some of these on my YouTube channel: https://www.youtube.com/user/newrulesofposture.

In many instances, you'll find relief for shoulder tension at the other end of the line—in the hands. The following section pursues this goal.

Eyes in your Elbows

As mentioned in chapter 3, most of our mundane daily tasks involve small motions of the arms and hands in front of the torso. In general, the elbows are flexed at more or less a 90-degree angle. This pattern of tension affects the tensegrity of the entire body, and a remnant of such tension often remains, even when the elbows are extended.

It is useful to imagine eyes in your elbows, similar to the ones in your hands, feet, and spine. A habit of chronic elbow flexion corresponds to elbow eyes that are squinting.

The following meditation helps you observe the extent of your unconscious arm tension. It also invites you to feel the way ease in your elbows contributes to your sense of wholeness.

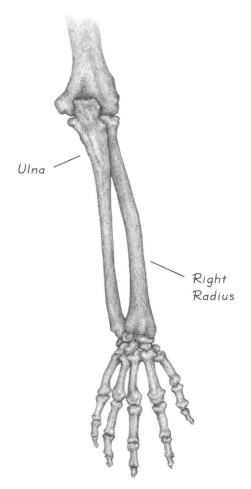

Ulna

Right Radius

The image shows the back of the right forearm with palm facing forward. For the palm to face back requires inward rotation of the radius around the ulna. Our human gestures of giving and receiving depend on freedom of movement of the radius bone. Habitual tension in the myofascia of the forearm restricts the rotation of the radius.

PRACTICE

Preparation for Arms Meditation

🔊 Practice 57 - Preparation for Arms Meditation

Begin by noticing the way your arms feel as they rest by your sides when you are in a standing position.

Then sit comfortably, either on the ground or on a chair. Be sure that your pelvis is inclined slightly forward. The twelve o'clock of your sacrum is a hair's breadth forward of your six o'clock. Be aware of the spaciousness of your pelvic floor. The slight forward inclination of your pelvis supports a gentle lumbar curve, and this in turn supports the uplift of your chest and throat. Relax your throat and jaw and recall the width of your upper palate. Check in with your midline.

Now become aware of your shoulder blades and let them slide down along the back of your body. Notice that your shoulder blades move a little as you breathe. They glide apart as your rib cage expands, and rest down along your back when you exhale.

Rest your palms on your thighs with your upper arms parallel to your torso. Be aware of the weight of your elbows. Notice whether one elbow feels lighter than the other. Spend an extra moment letting that elbow grow heavier. Sensing the weight of your elbows helps relax your shoulders.

PRACTICE

Arms Meditation

🔊 Practice 58 - Arms Meditation

Sit comfortably with your palms resting on your thighs. Sense your fascial breathing. Feel your skin surface expanding into the space as you breathe in. As you exhale, surrender the weight of your pelvis and leg bones to the ground. Feel the gentle swelling and shrinking of your breathing motion in your calves, in the soles of your feet, and between your toes.

Feel the gentle opening of your spinal drawers each time you inhale. Notice the increasing width between your armpits as your upper chest spreads.

Each time you exhale, let your shoulder blades and elbows renew their heaviness. Become aware of the weight of your hands on your upper thighs. Their weight makes a faint imprint in the fascia of your thighs.

Feel your fascial breathing in your hands. Each time you inhale, imagine the creases on your palms spreading apart from each other. As you exhale, the skin on your palms subtly shrinks.

Breathing in again, you can imagine your hands filling with air. Exhaling, you can sense the weight of the bones in your wrists and palms, and all the little bones in your fingers.

Bring your attention to your forearms. Notice the sensations of fascial breathing in the space between the two bones of each forearm. Inhaling, your palm lines spread, and your forearms soften and swell. Exhaling, you feel the weight of your hands and elbows.

Notice any distinction in how your two arms respond. Appreciate the difference without trying to change anything for now.

Appreciate the tensegral expansion of your breathing. Let every pore of your skin open and yield into the space. Let every bone find relationship to the ground.

Now stand and rest your arms along your sides. You may notice more space between your forearms and your wrists. More space between your forearms and your upper arms. If there were eyes in your elbows, they would be open. You may also notice more length along the front of your spine, as if the eyes in your spine have opened too. You might feel this in your throat, behind your heart, or through your diaphragm.

Application to Daily Living

Your arms are quintessentially expressive. They participate in your obviously expressive activities, like t'ai chi, tennis, or lovemaking, but they are also expressive in your everyday gestures. They convey your enthusiasm for whatever you're engaged in, and they communicate your resistance when that is the case.

Unconscious tension in your hands and arms has ramifications throughout your body. It is particularly prevalent among people who care for others—mothers and nurses, for example, or anyone who must be ready to act at a moment's notice. Upper extremity tension is also common among musicians, especially those who began playing an instrument as children. Musicians have a tendency to shape their bodies around their instruments when they play. Counterintuitive though it may be, learning to use the body tensegrally actually leads to better sound production.

Interoceptive awareness of your arms can be a profound experience. It gives you biofeedback about the degree to which your "doing" can interfere with your "being." Once you have deepened sensory awareness in your arms, you'll be able to interweave short sessions of this meditation into your daily activities. Dip into it, however briefly, after a period of computer work, preparing meals, or caring for someone. Run it in the background of your awareness while you're driving. You may even discover ways to rechoreograph the things you do so that your elbows, forearms, and hands don't constantly reassume compressive patterns.

As you apply the lens of your Body Mandala to your awareness of your arms, you may find that your pattern of arm tension has to do with letting go of agendas. Being present requires surrendering each recent moment and turning toward each next moment without anticipation. Only in the ever-fleeting present can we be wholly here.

> *O keep squeezing drops of the Sun from*
> *your prayers and work and music*
> *and from your companions' beautiful*
> *laughter, and from the most insignificant*
> *movements of your own holy body.*
>
> Excerpt from a longer poem by
> fourteenth-century Persian mystic Hafiz[6]

EPILOGUE

Expansion

I enjoy moving from a supported, adaptive, subtle place
where movement is not forced or owned
a place where touch goes beyond my physical being
a place where I am bigger than the me you see.
The eyes of my hands gaze beyond the star maps
of their creases to explore a world infinitely more
than the one where I previously existed.

SARAH TAYLOR*

Bridging to Real Life

When you bring your Body Mandala practice with you to the gym, trail, or yoga studio, your workout time includes recurring moments of midline awareness, wholeness, and perceptual tensegrity. Your exercise time is an opportunity to bring the introspective, detailed sensing of your Body Mandala journey into a context where movements are faster and more goal oriented. Practicing somatic presence while you move helps create a habit of being present during activity.

In doing this you establish a bridge to daily living, where much of your attention must be devoted outwardly and where many things take place quickly. The intention is to be ever more whole and present in your relationships to tasks, responsibilities, and deadlines, and in encounters with other people.

---

*Sarah, a Structural Integration practitioner and occupational therapist, wrote this poem during one of my classes in 2015.

Mandala Gates

For me, the gates of sensation and expression have generated more compelling insights into myself than have the gates of posture and movement. Posture and movement are easy to "fake," but your sensations and expressions are always truthful. For example, once you've recognized a sensation of closure in the back of your throat as a protective attitude, you have information you can use to change either your attitude or your current situation. Because sensations drive expression, familiarity with as many sensations as possible is beneficial. For this reason, the sensation gate is my go-to Body Mandala pathway.

In reality, the four gates of a Body Mandala are separate only in our minds. The mandala convention is a way to spread out your curriculum of self so you can approach it in bite-sized chunks. You are always traveling through all gates simultaneously.

Day by Day

By practicing sensations that support your experience of wholeness, you develop a repertoire of beneficial sensations. As those become familiar, harmful sensations—those indicating structural distortion, overly effortful movement, or perceptual limitation (like sagittal-plane living)—begin sticking out like sore thumbs. By expanding your sensory literacy, it becomes easier to listen to yourself in the language of sensation.

If body awareness is new to you, you may be tempted to try to feel everything at once. This will be discouraging. Because Body Mandala practice is a lifelong pursuit, there's time to take your time. Select a single sensation to focus on throughout a day. Only one. By noticing one, you'll likely notice others, but keep your focus on the one. Let it be that day's teacher. For example, you could breathe into the space between your forearm bones. (See the *Arms Meditation* in chapter 14.) When you tune into your interoception, you automatically tune into your fascial body as a whole. Your awareness triggers experience that is both fundamental and extraordinary.

Expressive Habits

To refine awareness of your expression, select a habit you know is counterproductive for your well-being, something presence-diminishing. This could be anything from negative self-talk ("I'm so stupid!") to chewing your cuticles. Then practice identifying the physical sensations that occur when you enter that habitual state—usually a combination of mental chatter and specific physical sensations. Then, again and again—you won't transform this overnight—offer yourself sensations you know will promote presence, sensations such as fascial breathing or back-space awareness. Over time you will map a new habit and develop a changed point of view.

For some time now, I've been studying the way I express myself when I'm late. (My ninety-five-year-old cousin claims that being late is a matter of failure to make decisions. But that's another conversation.) When I'm late, the tissues of my arms and shoulders feel brittle, my belly hardens, and my legs feel both sluggish and stiff. My upper spine curls down onto my heart, my head juts forward, and my eyes peer ahead as if I were wearing blinders. I add another layer to the knot at the top of my left shoulder. Perhaps I'm trying to make myself into a speeding bullet, like Superman. In a word, I become dense. Spatial awareness, of course, is the antidote for this. Being late becomes an opportunity to restore perceptual tensegrity when I notice myself in this state.

The other day I'd forgotten that Thursday morning traffic is worse than Friday mornings in Los Angeles, and I was about fifteen minutes behind schedule. But this time, upon feeling the familiar density, my eyes—on their own—moved to the far distance, to the low hills of Griffith Park. I sighed (I'd been holding my breath, of course) and noticed what a beautiful day it was.

That's the sweet reward of mandala practice—when a moment of habit recognition automatically triggers a perception that brings you into here, into now.

Being late might not be your thing, but I'm pretty sure you have an expressive pattern of a similar nature. A resistance or an urgency. Something that carves into your wholeness, crumples your midline, and takes you out of present time. Something worthy of study.

Orienting Perceptions

Until recently I was of the opinion that helping my clients and students feel and value the sensation of bodily weight was the most important somatic lesson I could share. But lately I've softened my opinion about this.

Yielding into our mothers' support as infants is a primary human impulse. It is somatic preparation for trust in terrestrial experience. As we mature, this primary yielding sensation develops into the capacity to relax. As you experienced in the *Rolling* practice (chapter 2), your body relaxes when you can allow yourself to receive support from the ground.

I firmly believed that restoring the capacity to yield was the foundational element in the development of somatic presence. It's the first "sensation" offered in this book. Perhaps I've been biased in this direction because of loyalty to Ida Rolf's message that "gravity is the therapist."[1]

Those of us who live in the sagittal plane must constantly renew awareness of our surroundings to keep from being confined by habitually narrowed spatial maps. For some of us, restoring panoramic spatial awareness may be a necessary precursor to the capacity to yield. In other words, we might need to broaden our horizons before we can rest easy.

At a certain point in your somatic self-study, the sensation of yielding no longer applies exclusively to the ground. In the moments when you experience yourself as a biotensegrity creature, you begin to realize that you can yield into your spatial surroundings. When you occupy your full bodily self, being present becomes a yielding—a resting in contact with the people, objects, and situations that comprise your present situation.

Being Present in the World

Modern living is complicated, and our world seems unlikely to become a more serene place anytime soon. What does it mean to be present amid the escalating hazards and pressures of the contemporary world?

The Digital Age appears to be sweeping aside the need for embodiment. Interacting with screens and pressing buttons, we require minimal bodily activity to make a day's journey. The semi-robotic use of our bodies makes dystopian films about humans being replaced by robots seem increasingly less far-fetched. The big-screen robots, you'll have noticed, are constructed using the compression model of the body with hinges, levers, and pulleys.

Body Mandala practice helps us remember that we are organisms rather than mechanisms. Deeply sensing our aliveness reminds us of our vulnerability. Biology entails mortality. Acknowledging our organismic natures changes how we relate to each other and how we perceive the world at large. This is a softer view, a slower pace. And a difficult choice at times.

Being present in the moment is, I believe, a natural human endowment and is both physiologically and evolutionarily necessary. Although presence incorporates inner stillness, it doesn't equate with absence of motion. To the contrary, there are times when presence must involve passionate action.

Your embodied presence in the midst of whatever is going on can help you assess your right next moves. Embodiment becomes an internal compass that directs you to the best way to respond to an immediate situation. It's a beat of inner quiet, a moment of global perspective in the midst of personal activity. It is the life within your life.

I hope *Body Mandala* has increased your capacity to listen to your body and to find value in what you hear. I hope you will discover the practicality of such listening. Body awareness is, of course, essential to improving posture, the hook for many readers who picked up this book. But beyond posture, somatic literacy can help you replace anxiety with calm, frustration with patience, and anger at another with grounded communication. Most of all, I hope it helps you to more often feel fully present during the precious mundane moments of your life.

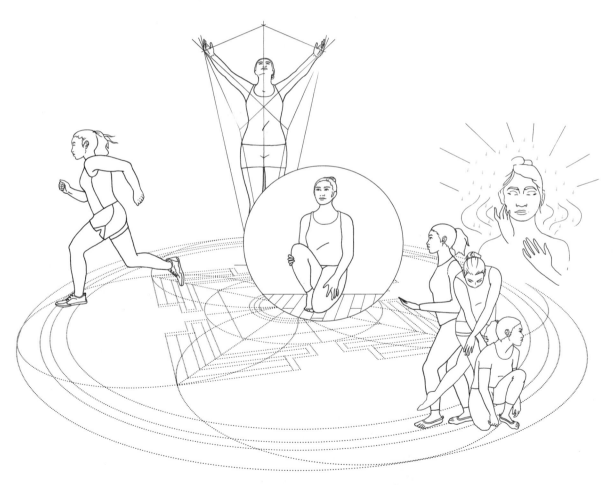

Like Tibetan sand mandalas, our bodies, too, will be swept away.
It is said that the depth of the journey will lighten the sweeping.

REFLECTION
A Work in Progress

Here's what I can tell you about my own Body Mandala journey to date: With respect to the "body reading" in the early pages of this book, the front and back halves of my body are well-balanced most of the time. I've been privileged to be involved with Rolfing Structural Integration for the past fifty years. I've taught its principles, written about it, and given and received many bodywork sessions. Something has come of that. My midline, conceived as a vertical gravitational symbol, is straight. But straightness isn't the whole story. A midline, you remember, is a perceptual activity rather than a location or position. It's a manifestation of dynamic perceptual tensegrity. In the thick of things, perceptions change. Sometimes my perceptions are tensegral; sometimes, not so much.

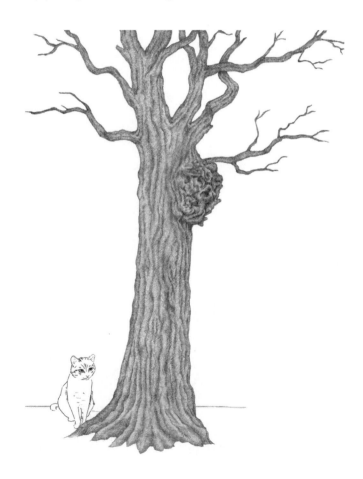

On off-days, my midline buckles behind my diaphragm. The disconnection there can express sorrow, anxiety, mental exhaustion, or plain old fatigue. Fascial breathing, when I remember it, tips the balance toward wholeness, where I'm better able to weather storms. Restoring midline polarity gives me perspective on my choices. Lately, however, I've exacerbated the buckling pattern by burrowing like a mole in my single-minded intention to share this book with you. Like anyone, I often take three steps forward and two back.

Regarding my structural organization, I don't know which comes first—whether my tensegrity tower leans to the left because of an imbalanced foundation, or whether the wincing impulse in my left armpit cascades down through my torso to the ground. But I no longer think it matters whether I discover the genesis of my shoulder pattern. These days, instead of seeing the pattern as a problem, I've come to regard it as a teacher—my interior sensei.

Not long ago I became upset during a transitional period in an organization of which I'm a member. One morning I decided to ask my body for a "reading" of my relationship to the situation. I've done this sort of thing for years, putting my interoception to work by letting my body become a divining rod. I frame my questions so as to receive a comparison between my current point of view and one that might be better for myself or for others. I figure there's a good chance the world at large, perhaps the universe and life itself, is organized according to the same tensional integrity that organizes bodies. So, by tuning into my body, I may get an indication about the best way to relate to the wider scheme of things. It's a way to summon my intuition.

The first step was to let my breathing settle, to become as present as I could. I let my mind yield into a state of not knowing. Then I asked the first question—in this case, "How am I viewing the communal situation?" A beat later my body felt like it was going to explode. I was holding my breath, bearing down in my gut, squeezing my lips and eyes, balling my hands into fists. Had there been steam coming out of my ears, it would have completed the cartoon-like image of personal fury. I'd had no idea I was *that* upset. And yet, I'd been waking up most mornings with headaches, a symptom that years ago had been associated with hypertension. Was I re-creating that now?

I moved around a bit, stretching and yawning, to free my mind and body of the first question. Then, standing relaxed, I asked the second: "How can I participate in this situation in a way that benefits myself and others?" My mind stilled.

After a few moments I "came to" with my left arm thrust to the side, palm outward, in a "stop" gesture. My right hand was placed over my heart. My feet were planted, my breathing steady. I seemed to be setting a boundary and remembering my center. Not bad advice for *any* situation.

My left shoulder and arm—whose tensions I've regarded as a minor disability—was showing me how to maintain my integrity. My weird postural habit—my wincing, weakness, and distortion—is also my sensitivity. It's a window to my inner self. It's good to tend to my shoulder, to stretch and strengthen it, to treat it to a massage. But I don't have to *perfect* it.

Like a burl in an old oak, it's a site of experience and wisdom.

ACKNOWLEDGMENTS

My immense gratitude goes to Hubert Godard for his insight into the degree to which our perceptions affect bodily form and function. Huge appreciation to my colleagues Robert Schleip and Thomas Myers for their dedication to bringing an understanding of fascia to mainstream health consciousness, and to Jean-Claude Guimberteau for generously allowing me to include his images of living fascia. My thanks also to Dunya Dianne McPherson for her insight into somatic contemplation and to Phillip Beach for teaching me *The Leonardos*.

I now know that *writing* a book is the "easy" part. Without the help of the following people, *Body Mandala* would have languished in my computer. Artists David Santa Maria and Joanna Skumanich worked long hours to make my words come alive with images—I'm still awed and delighted by their results. Artistic director, Harmony Ellington, went many extra miles to make the book's first edition feel good and look beautiful. Leslie Schwartz kept me from making assumptions and guided my storytelling. My colleagues Stacy Barrows, Diane Dalbey, Juan David Velez, and Michael Polon read the manuscript for accuracy and readability. The unflappable Ian Campbell, DP, patiently shot the video, Eric Podnar cheerfully recorded the hours and hours of audio, and Jason Adam designed the exquisite layout for the first edition. Aaron Bitz created the animations in chapters 9 and 10, Wina Gondokusumo modeled for the line drawings, and Danielle Owens-Reid and Julia Nunes were my expert crowdfunding guides. Thank you all so very much.

Much gratitude to the staff at Inner Traditions • Bear & Company, especially Jon Graham, for once again welcoming me and my book. It feels like coming home. Special thanks to my project editor, Kayla Toher, for her enthusiastic support and attention to detail.

I am also grateful to all my students for teaching me how to teach and for showing me what people need to know about human movement. My everlasting appreciation goes to the generous Kickstarter supporters who made production of the first edition possible.

To the memory of Ida P. Rolf for her contribution to the understanding of human bodies.

To the memory of Muhammad Subuh Sumohadiwidjojo for the gift of embodied spirituality.

GLOSSARY

Anal triangle of pelvic floor. The area between your two sit bones and your tailbone.

Anterior fontanelle. One of two main areas on an infant's head where bone formation is incomplete. These so-called "soft spots" are covered with fibrous connective tissue.

Atlanto-occipital joint. A juncture where two small bumps on the base of your skull fit into two shallow divots in your top neck vertebra. The joint is located right behind the top of your throat.

Biotensegrity. A scientific inquiry that applies the concept of tensegrity or tensional integrity to the study of all biologic organisms.

Body Image. Largely conscious, though sometimes unconscious, *opinion* about your body. It's how you see yourself in the world, and how you believe other people regard your body. Brain maps that create body image are linked through parts of the brain that store personal memory, social and cultural attitudes, expectations, beliefs, and emotions.

Body Schema. The felt experience of your body constructed by the maps in your brain. Built from the interaction of touch, vision, balance, hearing, spatial awareness, awareness of the positioning of your limbs, and of sensations inside your body, it's linked to the deep brain structures that manage survival.

Bregma. The place on the top of the head where the coronal and sagittal sutures come together when the anterior fontanelle closes.

Cervical. Refers to the neck or to the seven neck vertebrae.

Chronic hyperventilation syndrome. The tendency to take in more air than the body needs. Such "over-breathing" can result in a host of symptoms including lightheadedness, aching muscles, heart palpitations, chest pain, upset stomach, irritable bowel syndrome, sleeplessness, anxiety, depression, and more.

Coronal Plane. A vertical plane that divides the body into front and back. Also called "frontal plane."

Coupled motion of the spine. A combination of side-bending with simultaneous rotation of the spine.

Dorsiflexion. Movement at the ankle that decreases the angle between the top of the foot and the shin.

Embodiment. Term indicating body-mind connection through the body's perceptual capacity to influence human movement and behavior.

Enteric nervous system. Network of neurons governing the function of the gastrointestinal system.

Extension. A straightening movement that increases the angle between body parts. Straightening or backward bending of the spine. Opposite of flexion.

Exteroception. A type of proprioception that pertains to reception of stimuli through the traditional five senses—vision, touch, hearing, taste, and smell.

Exteroceptors. Sense receptors that give you information about the outside world, including vision, hearing, the balance system in your inner ears, and your tactile sense.

Fascia. A continuous gel-like yet fibrous medium that envelops, permeates, and interconnects all body structures, from the sheath that contains the body as a whole to the membranes that surround every nerve.

Feldenkrais Method. A gentle and effective system of movement rehabilitation based on targeted awareness to promote brain plasticity while learning optimal body organization.

Flexion. A bending or folding movement that narrows the angle between body parts. Forward bending of the spine. Opposite of extension.

Focusing. A method of working with the body's felt sense, developed by philosopher and psychotherapist Eugene Gendlin.

Foveal Vision. Sharp, central vision necessary for activities requiring visual detail. Contrasted with *peripheral vision,* which is outside the center of your gaze.

Horizontal plane. Relating to the horizon, perpendicular to the body's central vertical line.

Ideokinesis. A method of improving posture and movement through guided imagery.

Ilia. Plural of *ilium.* The broad bones forming the upper part of each side of the pelvis.

Insula, insular cortex. A region deep within the cerebral cortex that provides feedback about physical needs and well-being. By mapping visceral states associated with emotional experience, the insula plays a part in emotional processes, in empathy, and in consciousness.

Interoception. The capacity to sense yourself within your body. Interoceptive sensations include pain, tickle, hunger, thirst, taste, sexual arousal, pleasurable touch, and the sense of interior spaciousness.

Kyphosis. Indicates the normal forward curve or slight flexion of your thoracic spine.

Lordosis. Indicates the normal backward curve or slight extension of your lower back and neck.

Lumbar. Refers to the lower back, or to the five vertebrae of the lower spine.

Malleoli. The rounded protuberances at the bottom of the tibia and fibula that define the ankle joint.

Mechanotransduction. The process by which the mechanical forces transmitted through your body are converted into chemical changes within your cells.

Micromovement. Tiny movements of the body that enhance body awareness and sensory literacy.

Mirror Neurons. A network of brain cells that provides an internal somatic mimicry of the actions we notice in other people.

Movement Meditation. Movement meditation involves moving your body in improvisational ways, often with eyes closed, while maintaining a specific focus of awareness such as breathing.

Myofascia. Term used to indicate fascia that encompasses the muscles.

Neglected space. A region of peripersonal space where perception is diminished.

Neutral lumbar curve. The normal slight extension of the lumbar vertebrae.

Pandiculation. Involuntary whole body stretching that accompanies transitions between sleeping and waking.

Pelvic floor. The group of muscles that enclose the bottom of the pelvis, surround the urethra, vagina, and anus, and support the pelvic organs (bladder, uterus, and rectum).

Perceptual tensegrity. Balanced orientation to both the ground and the spatial environment. Supports internal body expansion, efficient and graceful coordination, and being present in the moment.

Perineal body. A fibrous fascial node formed by the interweaving of nine muscles that form the pelvic floor.

Perineal point. The author's informal coinage for the anatomical term *perineal body.*

Peripersonal space. Term used by neuroscientists to refer to the brain's multisensory representation of the space immediately surrounding the body.

Phasic. A type of muscular response. Phasic muscles are equipped, through their relationships with the circulatory, nervous, and connective tissue systems, to perform strong, short bursts of activity.

Plantar flex. To move the foot away from the shin, opening the angle at the ankle joint.

Postural Sway. A normal wavering of the body as your nerves, muscles, and fascia negotiate upright balance.

Pranayama. A yogic breathing discipline that has been shown to raise vagal tone and reduce the production of stress hormones.

Primitive Streak. A seam that appears in embryonic tissue fifteen days after conception, thought by many osteopaths to be the genesis of the body's energetic midline and life force.

Pronation. The natural inward turning movement of the foot around its midline.

Proprioception. Sensory input from your muscles, tendons, and joints, along with input from the balancing system in your inner ears, that informs you about the location of your body parts relative to one another. It lets you feel the shape of your body in the space around you and tells you how much effort is needed to position yourself and to move.

Rami. Plural of *ramus.* Curved branches of bone that connect the pubic bone to the two sit bones at the base of the pelvis. They form the bony boundary of the pelvic floor muscles.

Sacroiliac joints. Joints between the sacrum and ilia. Normal walking entails a minute amount of rotation at this joint.

Sacrum. The triangular-shaped bone wedged between the two *ilia.* Forms the back of the pelvic basin and the base of the spine.

Sagittal. A vertical plane that divides the body into right and left sides. Forward movement occurs in the sagittal plane.

Somatic. Comes from the Greek root word *soma,* meaning "body." In contemporary usage it has come to mean the sentient or feeling body.

Spinal discs. Spacers between the vertebrae. Formed of fibrocartilage (a type of fascia), spinal discs allow movement of the vertebrae and act as shock absorbers. Also called "intervertebral discs."

Supination. The natural outward turning movement of the foot around its midline.

Temporomandibular joint. The joint between the lower jawbone (*mandible*) and the *temporal* bone on the side of the head. Enables opening and closing of the mouth.

Tensegral expansion. Describes open and expanded bodily shape and movement. Joints are decompressed and fascial tensions are adjusted so that all elements in the biotensegrity body are participating.

Tensegrity. The integrity of a structure in which compression elements (such as bones) are supported by the balance of tensions through the continuous network (such as fascia) in which they are suspended.

Thoracic. Refers to the upper and middle spine, specifically the vertebrae of the rib cage.

Thoracic aperture. The opening at the top of the rib cage. Also known as "thoracic inlet."

Thoracic inlet. The opening at the top of the rib cage through which pass a group of blood vessels and nerves that relay messages between your brain and your hand and arm. Sometimes called the thoracic outlet.

Tibia. The larger of two bones of the lower leg. Its upper end forms a plateau on which the thigh rests. At the bottom it has a rounded protuberance (*malleolus*) that hugs the inside of the ankle.

Tibial tuberosities. Small bulges at the top front of the shinbone (*tibia*), below the knee joint. Called "shin points" in this book.

Tonic. A type of muscular response. Tonic muscles are equipped, through their relationships with the circulatory, nervous, and connective tissue systems, to be capable of sustained contraction.

Transversus abdominus. A deep, horizontally oriented muscle layer that surrounds and contains the abdomen.

Uvula. A flap of connective tissue that projects from the hard palate at the back of the throat. Helps close the throat during swallowing to prevent food from entering the nasal cavity. The uvula is located directly in front of your topmost neck vertebra.

Vagus nerve. Extensive neural pathway that connects your brain, heart, and gut. Affects the functioning of all the organs it touches and is associated with positive emotions.

Vector. A line of action. How far and in what direction your body as a whole, or a body part, has potential to move.

Vectoring. Guiding (an aircraft, for example) by means of radio communication according to vectors. With respect to the body: initiating a movement from a specific place in the body and along a specific line of action.

Viscera. Your internal organs, especially those contained in the abdominal and thoracic cavities.

Yield. Term used in this book to describe the primary act of relaxation. It implies the capacity to allow oneself to be supported by gravity.

NOTES

Introduction: What Is a Body Mandala?

1. Frank, "Tonic Function."
2. Farb et al., "Interoception, Contemplative Practice, and Health."

Chapter 1. Fascia: Organ of Embodiment

1. Guimberteau and Armstrong, *Architecture of Human Living Fascia*, 46.
2. Schleip et al., *Fascia*, 78.
3. Schleip et al., *Fascia*, 91.
4. Schleip et al., *Fascia*, 92.
5. Farb et al., "Interoception, Contemplative Practice, and Health."
6. Creswell et al., "Alterations in Resting-State Functional Connectivity Link Mindfulness Meditation with Reduced Interleukin-6."
7. Bellan, "The Strange Case of Interoception and Resilience."
8. Van der Wal, "The Architecture of the Connective Tissue in the Musculoskeletal System."
9. Schleip, "Episode #4—The Fascia Episode with Dr. Robert Schleip!"
10. Schleip et al., *Fascia*, 77.
11. Robert Schleip. Workshop notes taken by the author, January 2016.
12. Robert Schleip. Workshop notes taken by the author, January 2013.
13. Langevin, "Connective Tissue and Inflammation." Liberated Body website, accessed September 20, 2016. No longer available.
14. Still, *Philosophy and Mechanical Principles of Osteopathy*, 60.

Chapter 2. Grounding Your Experience

1. From Anita Barrows and Joanna Macy, trans., *Rilke's Book of Hours: Love Poems to God* (New York: Riverhead Books, 1996), 171.
2. Abram, "The Flesh of Language," in *The Spell of the Sensuous*, 73–92.
3. Blakeslee and Blakeslee, *The Body Has a Mind of Its Own,* 12.

Chapter 3. Sensing Space

1. Jordan, "Stanford Researchers Find Mental Health Prescription: Nature."
2. Brandt and Dieterich, "The Vestibular Cortex, Its Locations, Functions and Disorders."

Chapter 5. Exercises for Interoception

1. Roman et al., "Mathematical Analysis of the Flow of Hyaluronic Acid Around Fascia During Manual Therapy Motions."
2. Freeman, "What Happens in the Brain During an Orgasm?"
3. Porges, "The Polyvagal Theory."
4. Porges, "Steven Porges Conversation [with the Association for Comprehensive Energy Psychology]."

Chapter 7. Embodying Structure

1. Ingber, "Tensegrity and Mechanotransduction," 198–200.
2. As quoted by Feitus, *Ida Rolf Talks About Rolfing and Physical Reality*, 69.
3. Myers, "Spatial Medicine."
4. As quoted by Feitus, *Ida Rolf Talks About Rolfing and Physical Reality*, 86.
5. For a visual presentation of embryological development see "Human Embryology" on the *Bionalogy* website, October 13, 2016.

Chapter 8. Sentient Foundations

1. American Podiatric Medical Association, "New Survey Reveals Majority of Americans Suffer from Foot Pain," on the *Cision PR Newswire* website, May 19, 2014.
2. Beach, *Muscles and Meridians*, 3.
3. Robbins and Hanna, "Running-Related Injury Prevention through Barefoot Adaptations."
4. Oregon Research Institute. For more information, please reference "Oregon Study Confirms Health Benefits of Cobblestone Walking for Older Adults," on the *Science Daily* website, June 30, 2005.

Chapter 9. Your Spine Is Not a Column

1. Gracovetsky, *The Spinal Engine*, 9–17.
2. Doidge. *The Brain's Way of Healing*, 168.

Chapter 10. Tensegrity Tower

1. Richardson et al., *Therapeutic Exercise for Spinal Segmental Stabilization in Low Back Pain*.
2. Lederman, "The Myth of Core Stability."
3. Gendlin, *Focusing*.

Chapter 12. Embodying Tensegrity in Motion

1. Brody, "Distracted Walkers Pose Threat to Self and Others."
2. Ferrington and Rowe, "Cutaneous Mechanoreceptors and the Central Processing of Their Signals."
3. Bertolucci, "Pandiculation."
4. Ekelund et al., "Lack of Exercise Responsible for Twice as Many Deaths as Obesity."
5. Hausdorff et al., "The Power of Ageism on Physical Function of Older Persons."
6. Jordan, "Stanford Researchers Find Mental Health Prescription."

Chapter 13. Embodying Tensegrity in Stillness

1. O'Keefe, et al., "Organic Fitness: Physical Activity Consistent with Our Hunter-Gatherer Heritage."
2. Bowman, *Move Your DNA,* 105.
3. Olson, "Sitting Disease."

Chapter 14. Everyday Embodiment

1. Bowman, *Move Your DNA.*
2. O'Hare, "Exercise Is Good for Your Brain: Lifting Weights Could Make You More Intelligent and Stave off Dementia."
3. Robert Schleip. Workshop notes taken by the author, January 2016.
4. Robert Schleip. Workshop notes taken by the author, January 2016.
5. McDougall, *Born to Run.*
6. From Daniel Ladinsky, trans., *A Year with Hafiz: Daily Contemplations* (New York: Penguin Books, 2010), 339.

Epilogue

1. As quoted by Feitus, *Ida Rolf Talks About Rolfing and Physical Reality*, 121.

BIBLIOGRAPHY

Abram, David. "The Flesh of Language." In *The Spell of the Sensuous*. New York: Vintage Books, 1997.

American Podiatric Medical Association. "New Survey Reveals Majority of Americans Suffer from Foot Pain," on the Cision PR Newswire website. May 19, 2014.

Beach, Phillip. *Muscles and Meridians*. Edinburgh: Churchill Livingstone/Elsevier, 2010.

Bellan, Valeria. "The Strange Case of Interoception and Resilience." Body in Mind website. May 2016. No longer available.

Bertolucci, Luiz Fernando. "Pandiculation: Nature's Way of Maintaining the Functional Integrity of the Myofascial System?" *Journal of Bodywork and Movement Therapies* 15, no. 3 (July 2011): 268–80.

Blakeslee, Sandra, and Matthew Blakeslee. *The Body Has a Mind of Its Own*. New York: Random House, 2007.

Bond, Mary. *The New Rules of Posture: How to Sit, Stand, and Move in the Modern World*. Rochester, Vt.: Healing Arts Press, 2006.

Bowman, Katy. *Move Your DNA*. Carlsborg, Wash.: Priopriometrics Press, 2014.

Brandt, Thomas, and Marianne Dieterich. "The Vestibular Cortex, Its Locations, Functions and Disorders." *Annals of the New York Academy of Sciences,* no. 871 (1999): 293–312.

Brody, Jane. "Distracted Walkers Pose Threat to Self and Others." *New York Times Well* blog. December 7, 2015.

Creswell, J. David, Adrienne A. Taren, Emily K. Lindsay, Carol M. Greco, Peter J. Gianaros, April Fairgrieve, and Anna L. Marsland, et al. "Alterations in Resting-State Functional Connectivity Link Mindfulness Meditation with Reduced Interleukin-6: A Randomized Controlled Trial." *Biological Psychiatry* (July 2015).

Doidge, Norman. *The Brain's Way of Healing*. New York: Penguin Random House, 2015.

Earls, James. *Born to Walk: Myofascial Efficiency and the Body in Movement*. Berkeley: North Atlantic Books, 2014.

Eaton, S. Boyd, Marjorie Shostak, and Melvin Konner. *The Paleolithic Prescription*. New York: Harper and Row, 1988.

Ekelund, Ulf, et al. "Lack of Exercise Responsible for Twice as Many Deaths as Obesity." University of Cambridge Research website. January 14, 2015.

Farb, Norman, Jennifer Daubenmier, C. Price, et al. "Interoception, Contemplative Practice, and Health." Frontiers in Psychology website. June 2015.

Feitus, Rosemary, ed. *Ida Rolf Talks About Rolfing and Physical Reality*. New York: HarperCollins, 1979.

Ferrington, D., and Mark Rowe. "Cutaneous Mechanoreceptors and the Central Processing of Their Signals: Implications for Proprioceptive Coding." In *Proprioception, Posture, and Emotion*, 56–69. Kensington, Australia: University of New South Wales, 1982.

Frank, Kevin, "Tonic Function—A Gravity Response Model for Rolfing Structural Integration." *Journal of the Rolf Institute* 23, no. 1 (1995): 12–20.

Freeman, Shanna. "What Happens in the Brain During an Orgasm?" HowStuffWorks website. October 7, 2008.

Gendlin, Eugene. *Focusing*. New York: Bantam Dell, 1978. (A revised edition 2nd edition was printed in 1982).

Gracovetsky, Serge. *The Spinal Engine*. Vienna: Springer-Verlag, 1988.

Guimberteau, Jean-Claude, and Colin Armstrong. *Architecture of Human Living Fascia*. Edinburgh: Handspring Publishing, 2015.

Hausdorff, J. M., et al. "The Power of Ageism on Physical Function of Older Persons: Reversibility of Age-Related Gait Changes." *Journal of the American Geriatric Society* 47, no. 11 (November 1999): 1346–49.

Ingber, Donald E. "Tensegrity and Mechanotransduction." *Journal of Bodywork and Movement Therapies* 12, no. 3 (2008): 198–200.

Jordan, Rob. "Stanford Researchers Find Mental Health Prescription: Nature." Stanford News website. June 30, 2015. No longer available.

Lederman, Eyal. "The Myth of Core Stability." *Journal of Bodywork and Movement Therapies,* no. 14 (2010): 84–98.

McDougall, Christopher. *Born to Run: A Hidden Tribe, Superathletes, and the Greatest Race the World Has Never Seen*. New York: Vintage Books, 2011.

Myers, Thomas. *Anatomy Trains*. Edinburgh: Churchill Livingstone, 2001.

———. "Spatial Medicine—A Call to 'Arms.'" *Journal of Bodywork and Movement Therapies,* no. 18 (2013): 94–98.

O'Hare, Ryan. "Exercise Is Good for Your Brain: Lifting Weights Could Make You More Intelligent and Stave off Dementia." *Daily Mail* website. October 24, 2016.

O'Keefe, James H., et al. "Organic Fitness: Physical Activity Consistent with Our Hunter-Gatherer Heritage." *The Physician and Sportsmedicine* 38, no. 4. (2010): 1–8.

Olson, Lindsay. "Sitting Disease: The Slow, Silent and Sedentary Killer of the American Workforce," on the *U.S. News* website. August 22, 2013.

Oregon Research Institute. "Oregon Study Confirms Health Benefits of Cobblestone Walking for Older Adults," on the *Science Daily* website. June 30, 2005.

Porges, Stephen W. "The Polyvagal Theory." Podcast posted on the Somatic Perspectives on Psychotherapy website. November 2011.

———. "Stephen Porges Conversation." Posted to Youtube by the Association for Comprehensive Energy Psychology. February 13, 2015.

Richardson, Carolyn, Gwendolen Jull, Paul Hodges, and Julie Hides. *Therapeutic Exercise for Spinal Segmental Stabilization in Low Back Pain: Scientific Basis and Clinical Approach.* Edinburgh: Churchill Livingstone, 1999.

Robbins, Steven E., and Adel M. Hanna. "Running-Related Injury Prevention through Barefoot Adaptations." *Medicine and Science in Sports and Exercise,* no. 19 (1987): 148–155.

Rolf, Ida P. *Structural Integration: Gravity, an Unexplored Factor in a More Human Use of Human Beings.* San Francisco: Guild for Structural Integration, 1962.

Roman, Max, Hans Chaudhry, Bruce Bukiet, Antonio Stecco, and Thomas W. Findley. "Mathematical Analysis of the Flow of Hyaluronic Acid Around Fascia During Manual Therapy Motions." *Journal of the American Osteopathic Association,* no. 113 (2013): 600–610.

Schleip, Robert. "Episode #4—The Fascia Episode with Dr. Robert Schleip!" BodyAlignPro Podcast. Posted to Youtube by Body Align Pro. September 30, 2017.

Schleip, Robert, et al. *Fascia—The Tensional Network of the Human Body.* Edinburgh: Elsevier, 2012.

Still, Andrew T. *The Philosophy and Mechanical Principles of Osteopathy.* Kansas City, Mo.: Hudson-Kimberly, 1902.

Van der Wal, Jaap. "The Architecture of the Connective Tissue in the Musculoskeletal System." *Fascia Research II,* edited by P. A. Huijing, et al. Munich: Elsevier, 2009.

INDEX

Page numbers in *italics* refer to illustrations.

ABOUT THE AUTHOR

Mary Bond has a master's degree in dance from UCLA and trained with Ida Rolf, Ph.D., as a Structural Integration practitioner. Formerly Chair of the Movement Faculty of the Dr. Ida Rolf Institute, Mary teaches workshops tailored to the needs and interests of various groups such as dancers, Pilates, yoga and fitness instructors, massage therapists, and people who sit for a living. Her articles have appeared in numerous health and fitness magazines and she hosts a popular blog at www.healyourposture.com.

Mary's first book, *Balancing Your Body: A Self-help Approach to Rolfing Movement,* was published in 1993 by Healing Arts Press. In it she offered a self-help version of Rolf Movement therapy. Her second book, *The New Rules of Posture,* presented developments in Rolf Movement education. It evolved out of Mary's wish to share the legacy of Ida Rolf with the general public. While this legacy includes the understanding of posture and movement, it also has philosophical implications. The deeper message is that the way we inhabit our bodies affects the ways in which we perceive the world and behave toward one another. Her 2012 video workshop, *Heal Your Posture,* further elucidates this message.